Monitoring the Critically Ill Patient

Second edition

Philip Jevon
RGN, BSc (Hon), PGCE, ENB 124
Resuscitation Officer/Clinical Skills Lead
Honorary Clinical Lecturer
Manor Hospital
Walsall
UK

AND

Beverley Ewens
RN, BSc (Hon), PGCE, ENB 100, PG Dip
Staff Development Nurse
Critical Care Unit
Joondalup Health Campus
Perth
Western Australia

CONSULTING EDITOR

Jagtar Singh Pooni
BSc (Hons) MRCP (UK) FRCA
Consultant in Anaesthesia and Intensive Care Medicine
New Cross Hospital
Wolverhampton
UK

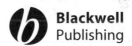

Blackwell
Publishing

WB 300

© 2002 by Blackwell Science Ltd, a Blackwell Publishing company
© 2007 by Blackwell Publishing

Blackwell Publishing editorial offices:
Blackwell Publishing Ltd, 9600 Garsington Road, Oxford OX4 2DQ, UK
Tel: +44 (0)1865 776868
Blackwell Publishing Inc., 350 Main Street, Malden, MA 02148-5020, USA
Tel: +1 781 388 8250
Blackwell Publishing Asia Pty Ltd, 550 Swanston Street, Carlton, Victoria
3053, Australia
Tel: +61 (0)3 8359 1011

First published 2002 by Blackwell Science Ltd
Second edition published 2007 by Blackwell Publishing Ltd

3 2008

Library of Congress Cataloging-in-Publication Data

Jevon, Philip.
Monitoring the critically ill patient /
Philip Jevon and Beverley Ewens. – 2nd ed.
p. ; cm. – (Essential clinical skills for nurses)
Includes bibliographical references and index.
ISBN 978-1-4051-4440-7 (pbk.: alk. paper)
1. Patient monitoring. 2. Critical care medicine.
I. Ewens, Beverley. II. Title. III. Series.
[DNLM: 1. Intensive Care–methods. 2. Monitoring, Physiologic–
methods. 3. Critical Illness. WX 218 J58m 2007]

RT48.55.M665 2007
616′. 028–dc22
2007009060

A catalogue record for this title is available from the British Library

Set in 9/11pt Palatino
by SNP Best-set Typesetter Ltd., Hong Kong
Printed and bound in Singapore
by Fabulous Printers Pte Ltd

For further information on Blackwell Publishing, visit our website:
www.blackwellnursing.com

From reviews of the first edition:

'. . . an excellent quick reference guide to all the different types of patient monitoring used in critical care. It will be useful for nurses working in acute wards and for junior nurses working in ICU and high-dependency units.'
Nursing Times

'. . . the compact nature of the book will make it a useful reference for those responsible for monitoring critically ill or potentially critically ill patients, where nursing care is delivered.'
Journal of Advanced Nursing

'This comprehensive book shows, in a nutshell, the most important issues needed for monitoring critically ill patients, not only in ICU but also in A&E settings. The authors were successful in writing this down in a clear and readable way, and it is logically presented . . . an ideal basis for advanced learning.'
Accident and Emergency Nursing

'. . . an invaluable text that will help to facilitate high quality care for the most vulnerable patients.'
British Journal of Resuscitation

Contents

Foreword

Advances in tertiary health care practices have resulted in an increasingly rapid turnover of patients in the hospital system. Patients are admitted later, discharged earlier and recuperate at home. As a direct consequence of this, patients within the hospital are of a much higher acuity than before. This has heightened the need for staff to rapidly and accurately assess and monitor the health status of patients in their care. Many hospitals have implemented early warning systems as a means of detection and management of patient deterioration. This is in response to recognised antecedents to deterioration which exist but are often not recognised in acute care settings. Accurate and appropriate monitoring with interpretation of the resulting data is the key to success in the management of these critical events.

The contributors to this book have extensive international critical care experience. The book will prove to be a valuable resource for registered nurses, student nurses and enrolled nurses practicing in critical care, high dependency units and the acute ward environment. It provides an invaluable tool for recognising and monitoring critically ill patients. The book encompasses the full range of patient monitoring from non-invasive through to invasive techniques and is therefore a suitable resource for both the novice and the expert practitioner.

This book builds upon the success of the first edition. The content has been updated to reflect current practice and includes two new chapters on recognition and management of the critically ill patient. These chapters detail the principles underlying early warning systems, medical emergency teams, and critical care outreach teams. Emphasis on the early recognition of the deteriorating patient, to facilitate prompt intervention and improve outcomes is an underlying philosophy of this text.

Alan Tulloch
RN, MSc Nursing
Lecturer
School of Nursing
Curtin University of Technology
Perth, West Australia.

Preface

Welcome to the second edition of *Monitoring the Critically Ill Patient*. This edition has been updated to reflect current developments in practice. A new chapter has been included on outreach, medical emergency teams (MET) and early warning scoring (EWS) systems. Highly dependent patients are currently and will be in the future, managed in ward areas with the support of outreach teams. We have indeed created a critical care unit without walls.

Nurses, whether they are working in intensive care units, high dependency areas or in wards, must possess the necessary knowledge and expertise to accurately and safely monitor critically ill patients. The early detection of problems, together with appropriate management, is paramount and will ultimately improve outcomes.

We hope this second edition continues to provide nurses with a valuable resource as they strive to deliver optimum standards of nursing care to these patients.

March 2007

Acknowledgements

The authors are grateful to:

- Jagtar Singh Pooni, Consultant in Anaesthesia and Intensive Care Medicine at New Cross Hospital, Wolverhampton, for his help with writing Chapters 4 and 14 and for kindly agreeing to be consultant editor for the book;
- John Hamilton and his staff at the Medical Photography Department at the Manor Hospital in Walsall for their assistance with photographs;
- Laerdal Medical for providing the ECG traces;
- Tim Simmonds, formally Senior Charge Nurse on ICU at the Manor Hospital in Walsall for his help with Chapter 11;
- Dee Cope, Nurse Specialist on Neuro ICU at University Hospital, Birmingham, for her help with Chapter 6;
- *Nursing Times* for granting us permission to reproduce material from an article we wrote for them;
- Cambridge University Press, Butterworth-Heinemann, Churchill Livingstone, Baillière Tindall, Routledge and Oxford University Press for kindly granting us permission to reproduce material from their publications.

Recognition and Management of the Critically Ill Patient

INTRODUCTION

Critically ill patients have a high morbidity and high mortality (Gwinnutt 2006). Prompt recognition and early appropriate management of patients who are at risk of being, or who are, critically ill, can help to prevent further deterioration and maximise the chances of recovery (Gwinnutt 2006). This proactive approach may negate the need for admission to the intensive care unit (ICU) and could reduce mortality and morbidity for those admitted at the appropriate time (McQuillan *et al.* 1998; McGloin *et al.* 1999; Young *et al.* 2003).

The aim of this chapter is to understand the recognition and management of the critically ill patient.

LEARNING OBJECTIVES

At the end of this chapter the reader will be able to:

❏ discuss the importance of prevention of in-hospital cardiopulmonary arrest
❏ list the clinical signs of critical illness
❏ discuss the role of outreach and medical emergency teams
❏ discuss the importance of staff training relating to the recognition of the critically ill patient

PREVENTION OF IN-HOSPITAL CARDIOPULMONARY ARREST

Survival to discharge from in-hospital cardiopulmonary arrest

In the UK, only 17% of patients who have an in-hospital cardiopulmonary arrest survive to discharge (Nolan *et al.* 2005). Most of these survivors will have received prompt and effective defibrillation for a monitored and witnessed ventricular fibrillation arrest (Fig. 1.1), caused by primary myocardial ischaemia (Resuscitation Council UK 2006). Survival to discharge in these patients is very good, even as high as 42% (Gwinnutt *et al.* 2000).

Unfortunately, most in-hospital cardiopulmonary arrests are caused by either asystole (Fig. 1.2) or pulseless electrical activity (PEA) (i.e. no pulse, but an ECG trace that would normally be expected to produce a cardiac output e.g. Fig. 1.3), both non-shockable rhythms are associated with a very poor outcome (Nolan *et al.* 2005). These arrests are usually not sudden and are not unpredictable: cardiopulmonary arrest usually presents as a final step in a sequence of progressive deterioration of the presenting illness, involving hypoxia and hypotension (Resuscitation Council UK 2006). These patients rarely survive to discharge; the only approach that is likely to be successful is prevention of the cardiopulmonary arrest (Gwinnutt 2006). For this prevention strategy to be successful, recognition and effective treatment of patients at risk of cardiopulmonary arrest are paramount. This may prevent some cardiac arrests, deaths and unanticipated ICU admissions (Nolan *et al.* 2005). The ACADEMIA study demonstrated that antecedents were present in 79% of cardiopulmonary arrests, 55% of deaths and 54% of unanticipated ICU admissions (Kause *et al.* 2004).

Sub-optimal critical care

Studies have shown that the care of critically ill inpatients in the UK is frequently sub-optimal (McQuillan *et al.* 1998; McGloin *et al.* 1999). Junior staff frequently fail to recognise and appreciate the severity of illness and when therapeutic interventions are implemented these have often been delayed or are inappropriate. The management of deteriorating inpatients is a significant problem, particularly at night and at weekends, when responsibilities for these patients usually falls to the acute take team whose main focus is on a rising tide of new admissions (Baudouin & Evans 2002).

In a confidential inquiry into quality of care before admission to ICU, two external reviewers assessed the quality of care in 100 consecutive admissions to ICU (McQuillan *et al.* 1998):

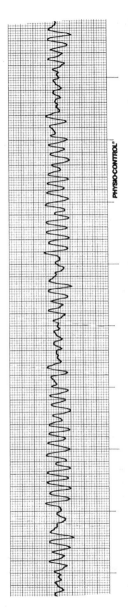

Fig. 1.1 Ventricular fibrillation (coarse).

PHYSIO-CONTROL®

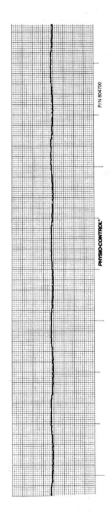

Fig. 1.2 Asystole.

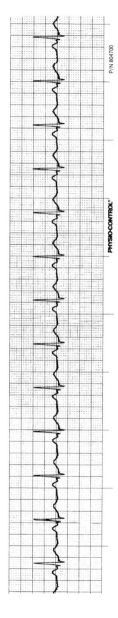

Fig. 1.3 Pulseless electrical activity (PEA)/Sinus rhythm.

- 20 patients were deemed to have been well managed and 54 to have received sub-optimal management, with disagreement about the remainder.
- Case mix and severity were similar between the groups, but ICU mortality was worse in those who both reviewers agreed received sub-optimal care prior to ICU admission (48% compared with 25% in the well managed group).
- Admission to ICU was considered late in 37 patients in the sub-optimal group. Overall, a minimum of 4.5% and a maximum of 41% of admissions were considered potentially avoidable.
- Sub-optimal care contributed to morbidity or mortality in most instances.
- The main causes of sub-optimal care were failure of organisation, lack of knowledge, failure to appreciate clinical urgency, lack of supervision and failure to seek advice.

Even more disturbingly, studies of events leading to 'unexpected' in-hospital cardiac arrest indicate that many patients have clearly recorded evidence of marked physiological deterioration prior to the event, without appropriate action being taken in many cases (Schein *et al*. 1990; Franklin & Mathew 1994).

Deficiencies in critical care frequently involve simple aspects of care, e.g. failure to recognise and effectively treat abnormalities of the patient's airway, breathing and circulation, incorrect use of oxygen therapy, failure to monitor the patient, failure to ask for help from senior colleagues, ineffective communication, lack of teamwork and failure to use treatment limitation plans (McQuillan *et al*. 1998; Hodgetts *et al*. 2002).

The ward nurse is uniquely based to recognise that the patient is starting to deteriorate and to alert the appropriate help (Adam & Osborne 2005). However, response times by ward staff are unacceptably variable (Rich 1999).

Strategies to prevent in-hospital cardiac arrest

Nolan *et al*. (2005) suggest that the following strategies may help to prevent avoidable in-hospital cardiopulmonary arrests:

- Provide care for patients who are critically ill or at risk of clinical deterioration in appropriate areas, with the level of care provided matched to the level of patient sickness.

- Critically ill patients need regular observations: match the frequency and type of observations to the severity of illness or the likelihood of clinical deterioration and cardiopulmonary arrest. Often only simple vital sign observations (pulse, blood pressure, respiratory rate) are needed.
- Use an early warning score (EWS) system to identify patients who are critically ill and/or at risk of clinical deterioration and cardiopulmonary arrest.
- Use a patient charting system that enables the regular measurement and recording of EWS.
- Have a clear and specific policy that requires a clinical response to EWS systems. This should include advice on the further clinical management of the patient and the specific responsibilities of medical and nursing staff.
- The hospital should have a clearly identified response to critical illness. This may include a designated outreach service or resuscitation team (e.g. medical emergency team (MET)) capable of responding to acute clinical crises identified by clinical triggers or other indicators. This service must be available 24 hours per day.
- Train all clinical staff in the recognition, monitoring and management of the critically ill patient. Include advice on clinical management while awaiting the arrival of more experienced staff.
- Identify patients for whom cardiopulmonary arrest is an anticipated terminal event and in whom cardiopulmonary resuscitation (CPR) is inappropriate, and patients who do not wish to be treated with CPR. Hospitals should have a DNAR (do not attempt resuscitation) policy, based on national guidance, which is understood by all clinical staff.
- Ensure accurate audit of cardiac arrest, 'false arrest', unexpected deaths and unanticipated ICU admissions using common datasets. Audit also the antecedents and clinical response to these events.

CLINICAL SIGNS OF CRITICAL ILLNESS
The clinical signs of critical illness and deterioration are usually similar regardless of the underlying cause, because they reflect compromise of the respiratory, cardiovascular and

neurological functions (Nolan *et al.* 2005). These clinical signs are commonly:

- tachypnoea
- tachycardia
- hypotension
- altered conscious level (e.g. lethargy, confusion, restlessness or falling level of consciousness)

(Resuscitation Council UK 2006)

Tachypnoea, a particularly important indicator of an at-risk patient (Goldhill *et al.* 1999), is the most common abnormality found in critical illness (Goldhill & McNarry, 2004). Fieselmann *et al.* (1993) found that a raised respiratory rate (>27/minute) occurred in 54% of patients in the 72 hours preceding cardiac arrest, most of which occurred at 72 hours prior to the event.

The identification of abnormal clinical signs (together with the patient's history, examination and appropriate investigations) is central to objectively identifying patients who are at risk of deterioration (Buist *et al.* 1999). However, these clinical signs of deterioration are often subtle and can go unnoticed. It is therefore essential that tools, which reflect best evidence, are developed and available to aid the practitioner to identify signs of deterioration. Ultimately this may prevent adverse events and improve patient outcomes.

EARLY WARNING SCORES AND CALLING CRITERIA

Many hospitals now use EWS or calling criteria systems to help in the early detection of critical illness (Goldhill *et al.* 1999; Hodgetts *et al.* 2002; Subbe *et al.* 2003; Buist *et al.* 2004). Their sensitivity, specificity and reliability to predict clinical outcomes has yet to be convincingly proven (Cuthbertson 2003; Parr 2004). However, there is a sound rationale for using these systems to identify sick patients early (Nolan *et al.* 2005).

Although there are no data demonstrating the best system, the EWS approach may be preferable because it tracks changes in physiology and warns of impending physiological collapse, while the calling criteria approach is only triggered if an extreme physiological value is recorded (Nolan *et al.* 2005).

Early warning scores

Comprehensive Critical Care (Department of Health, 2000) recommended the widespread implementation of EWS systems and outreach services. The EWS systems have been developed as a tool to enable ward staff to combine their regular observations to produce an aggregate physiological score (Sharpley & Holden 2004). They are based upon the premise that there is a common physiological pathway of deterioration in the critically ill patient, which can be detected by simple ward-based observations (Goldhill 2001).

A weighted score is attached to a combination of blood pressure, pulse, respiratory rate, oxygen saturations, temperature, urine output and simplified level of consciousness (AVPU) (Fig. 1.4). Once a certain score is reached, nursing and other paramedical staff must then alert the designated expert help following local protocols. Escalation policies are put in place whereby a failure to improve (or to receive prompt help) results in the immediate contact of more senior members (including consultant staff) (Baudouin & Evans 2002). Clear guidelines should be drawn up to guide the nurse when and whom to contact for help (Fig. 1.5).

Each hospital should have a track and trigger system that allows rapid detection of the signs of early clinical deterioration and an early and appropriate response (NCEPOD, 2005). These track and trigger systems should be robust, should cover all inpatients and should be linked to a response team that is appropriately skilled to assess and manage the clinical problems (NCEPOD, 2005). However, 27% of hospitals do not use an EWS system (NCEPOD, 2005).

- **A**lert
- Responds to **v**oice
- Responds to **p**ain
- **U**nconscious
  (Resuscitation Council UK 2006)

Fig. 1.4 Level of consciousness.

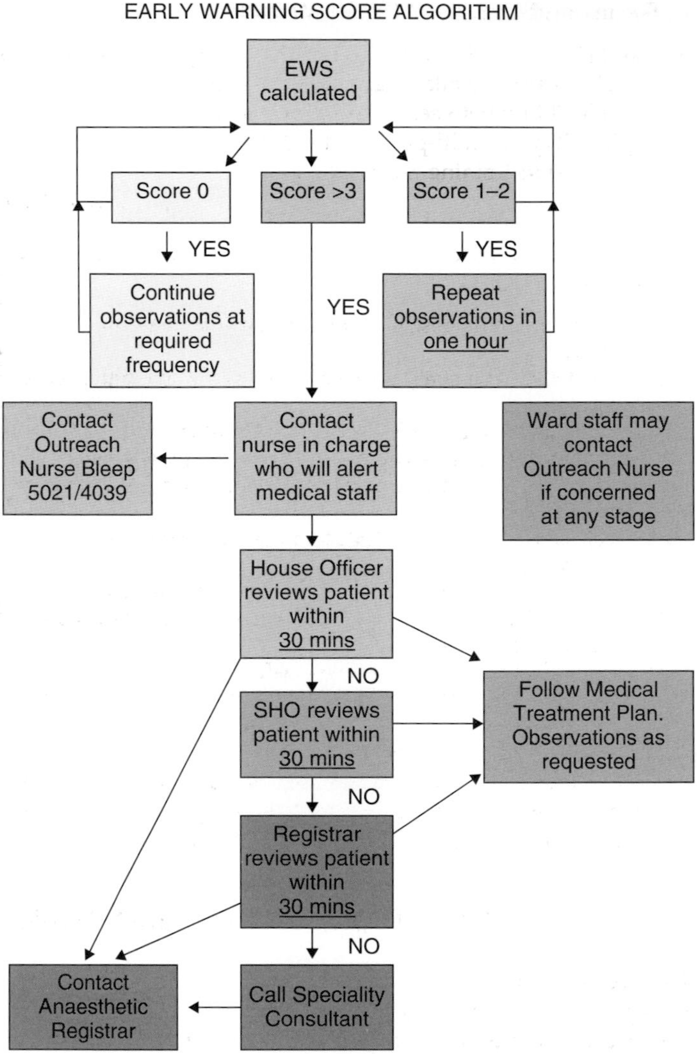

EARLY WARNING SCORE ALGORITHM

Fig. 1.5 Early warning score algorithm (Walsall Hospitals NHS Trust).

The main advantages of EWS systems are:

- simplicity: only the basic monitoring equipment is required (usually readily available on acute wards)
- reproducibility between different observers
- applicability to multi-professional team
- minimal staff training required

(Gwinnutt 2006)

Best practice – EWS

EWS score should be designed to reflect subtle changes in condition

EWS chart should be straightforward to use and unambiguous in its design

Implementation should be planned and coordinated

Extensive education strategy is needed prior to implementation

Specific guidelines should be attached to the EWS, e.g. who to call and when

EWS calling criteria can be adjusted for specific patients, e.g. chronic disease

Audit of EWS charts is carried out to assess completeness

Audit is carried out of specific incidents where calling criteria were not adhered to

There should be ongoing education of staff

Calling criteria systems

'Calling criteria' systems are based on routine observations, which activate a response when an extreme physiological value is reached (Lee *et al.* 1995; Goldhill *et al.* 1999).

ROLE OF OUTREACH AND MEDICAL EMERGENCY TEAMS

Outreach teams

Comprehensive Critical Care (Department of Health, 2000) recommended the development of outreach teams in all acute Trusts. They have been established in accordance with the 'intensive care without walls' philosophy as one aspect of the critical care service (Gwinnutt 2006). The objectives of outreach teams are to:

- avert ICU admissions by identifying patients who are deteriorating and either helping to prevent admission or ensuring that admission to a critical care bed happens in a timely manner to ensure best outcome
- enable ICU discharges by supporting both the continuing recovery of discharged patients on wards and after discharge from hospital
- share critical care skills with staff in wards and the community, ensuring enhancement of training opportunities and skills practice and using information gathered from the ward and community to improve critical care services for patients and relatives

(Department of Health 2000)

All acute Trusts should have a formal outreach service that is available 24 hours per day, seven days per week (NCEPOD, 2005). The composition of this service will vary from hospital to hospital but it should comprise of individuals with the skills and ability to recognise and manage the problems of critical illness (NCEPOD, 2005). Outreach services should not replace the role of traditional medical teams in the care of inpatients, but should be seen as complementary (NCEPOD, 2005).

Many outreach services are often not available on a 24-hour basis, however (NCEPOD, 2005). Some only provide cover for selected patients, e.g. following surgery (NCEPOD, 2005). Forty-four percent of hospitals do not even provide an outreach service (NCEPOD, 2005).

Despite widespread acceptance and intuitive belief in the benefit of outreach teams, there is a lack of evidence to support their use,

---

Best practice – outreach teams

Clear operational guidelines
Structured work practices
Ownership by senior Trust managers and clinicians
Clear lines of communication throughout the organisation
Strong links with other teams to share practice and disseminate ideas
Identify and address training needs in ward areas
Act as a resource and support for ward staff

---

there are national variations in their availability, there is no consensus about the ideal composition and there is no consensus regarding triggers to activate referral (Holder & Cuthbertson 2005).

Medical emergency teams
In some hospitals the cardiac arrest team, which has traditionally only been called once the patient has had a cardiopulmonary arrest, has been replaced by a MET (Nolan *et al.* 2005). The MET not only responds to patients in cardiopulmonary arrest, but also to those with acute physiological deterioration (Lee *et al.* 1995). METs were first developed in Australia in the 1990s where they are now commonplace. The MET approach demonstrates proactive and pre-emptive management of the patient at risk. The aim of a MET is to pre-empt deterioration and prevent adverse events (Lee *et al.* 1995; Goldhill *et al.* 1999; Bristow *et al.* 2000; Buist *et al.* 2002; Bellomo *et al.* 2003).

METs are reliant upon calling criteria (Table 1.1) whereupon the team will automatically be called. They will then assess and

Table 1.1 MET calling criteria, Joondalup Health Campus (reproduced by kind permission of Brendon Burns).

Acute changes in	Physiology
Airway	Threatened
Breathing	• RESPIRATORY ARREST • Respiratory rate <8 breaths/min • Respiratory rate >36 breaths/min • Pulse oximetry; saturation <90% despite oxygen administration
Circulation	• CARDIAC ARREST • Heart rate <40 beats/min • Heart rate >140 beats/min • Systolic blood pressure <90 mmHg
Neurology	• Sudden fall in level of consciousness • Fall of GCS >2 points
Urine output	• <50 ml total over 4 hours
OR	
Staff member is seriously concerned about the patient	

treat the patient as required with the explicit aim of preventing deterioration. Evidence is currently emerging exploring the efficacy of METs and improvement in outcomes. Members of the MET may include:

- experienced ICU nurse
- anaesthetist
- physician

Best practice – MET

Calling criteria should be evidence based
Staff must be aware of the MET calling criteria
MET calling criteria should be visible in all wards and departments
Staff should carry individual copies of MET calling criteria
Regular education sessions to update staff
MET education sessions on all staff orientation programmes
Audit of all MET calls to identify trends and deficiencies
Audit of cardiac arrests
Utilise data as part of learning needs analysis
Inappropriate MET calls should be dealt with sensitively so that staff
   are not discouraged to call MET in the future

CLASSIFICATION AND PROVISION OF CRITICAL CARE

'Critical care without walls'

Comprehensive Critical Care (Department of Health, 2000) recommended that critical care should be delivered, encapsulating the philosophy 'critical care without walls', i.e. the needs of the critically ill must be met, no matter where such patients are physically located within the hospital. Critical care should be mobile, offering advice, assistance and education outside the traditional confines of the ICU (Baudouin & Evans 2002).

Classification of critical care

Classification of critical care patients should focus on the level of care that individual patients require, regardless of their location (Department of Health, 2000). This approach sees a shift of emphasis away from defining patient needs in terms of hospital geography, e.g. ICU, high dependency unit (HDU) etc., and

Table 1.2 Classification of critical care patients (Department of Health, 2000).

Level	Description
Level 0	Patients whose needs may be met through normal ward care in an acute hospital
Level 1	Patients at risk of their condition deteriorating, or those recently relocated from higher levels of care, whose needs can be met on an acute ward with additional advice and support from the critical care team
Level 2	Patients requiring more detailed observation or intervention including support for a single failing system or post-operative care and those 'stepping down' from higher levels of care
Level 3	Patients requiring advanced respiratory support alone or basic respiratory support together with support of at least two organ systems. This level includes all complex patients requiring support for multi-organ failure

towards a classification system that describes escalating levels of care for individual patients, independent of their location within the hospital (Table 1.2) (Gwinnutt 2006).

The Intensive Care Society (2002) has provided more detailed explanations and definitions of the classification levels. These definitions facilitate the assessment and quantification of the hospital-wide demand for the different levels of care, removing geographical location from being the defining factor for patients accessing critical care (Adam & Osborne 2005).

Provision of critical care

ICU bed provision in the UK has historically been one of the lowest in the industrialised world (Edbrooke *et al.* 1999). Prior to the publication of Comprehensive Critical Care (Department of Health, 2000), only 2.6% of hospital beds were designated ICU beds, compared to 3.3% in Europe and 5–7% in North America (Baudouin & Evans 2002). The ICU bed capacity has now increased. In England, there are now 22% more beds catering for patients termed level 2 and level 3 dependency (Table 1.2) (Department of Health, 2000).

TRAINING HEALTHCARE STAFF

Several studies have demonstrated that both medical and nursing staff lack the necessary knowledge and skills in acute care (Nolan *et al.* 2005), e.g. lack of knowledge regarding oxygen therapy (Smith & Poplett 2002), pulse oximetry (Kruger *et al.* 1997) and fluid and electrolyte balance (Meek 2000). Senior medical staff's knowledge and skills may also be deficient. Healthcare staff rarely have the confidence to deal with acutely ill patients and often do not follow a systematic approach to assessing them. In addition, deficiencies in acute care often involve simple interventions, e.g. treating problems affecting airway, breathing and circulation (McQuillan *et al.* 1998). The combination of poor early recognition and lack of key skills in responding to acute deterioration probably contributes to poor patient outcome (Adam & Osborne 2005).

There have been several educational initiatives to improve multi-disciplinary knowledge, skills and attitudes concerning the management of the critically ill patient (Kause *et al.* 2004), some of which will now be described.

ALERT course

The ALERT (Acute Life-threatening Events – Recognition and Treatment) course was developed at Portsmouth University in 1999 with the aim of improving acute care of both 'at risk' and critically ill adult patients. It was specifically designed to address the anxieties and areas of perceived weakness in the management of the acutely ill patient, previously identified by ward nurses and pre-registration house officers. It has several aims:

- a reduction in avoidable cardiac arrests
- a reduction in avoidable hospital deaths
- a reduction in avoidable ICU admissions
- better recognition of the 'at risk' or acutely ill patient
- better clinical management of the 'at risk' or acutely ill patient
- better partnership and teamwork between healthcare professionals
- better written and verbal communication

A simple assessment and management system is described which can be used for ill patients with a wide range of underlying clinical conditions, both medical and surgical. The course is mainly designed to train pre-registration house officers and junior nurses. However, other staff groups, e.g. medical students, senior house officers and senior nurses may also find it helpful.

The 1-day ALERT course has been designed so that medical and nursing staff can train together using a common approach. It is designed on sound principles of adult education – active involvement, personal motivation, experience-centred learning, relevance to practice, regular feedback, clear goals and the use of reflective practice. For further information see www.port.ac.uk.

Advanced Trauma Life Support (ATLS) course

The 2.5-day ATLS course, developed by the American College of Surgeons in the 1980s, has now been adopted in over 30 countries worldwide. It teaches a simple systematic approach to the management of trauma patients, treating the most life-threatening injury. A highly interactive course, it combines lectures, discussions, interactive tutorials, skills teaching and simulated patient management scenarios (moulage). For further information: Royal College of Surgeons of England, tel – 020 7869 6309, email – atls@rcseng.ac.uk.

Advanced Life Support (ALS) course

The Resuscitation Council (UK) ALS course aims to teach the theory and practical skills to effectively manage cardiorespiratory arrest, peri-arrest situations and special circumstances. There is a big emphasis on prevention of cardiopulmonary arrest. The 2-day course comprises lectures, practical skill stations, workshops and assessments. Candidates are sent a course manual to read 4 weeks prior to the course. For further information see www.resus.org.uk.

Immediate Life Support (ILS) course

The ILS course is mainly designed to equip the first responder with the necessary skills to manage a cardiac arrest while awaiting the arrival of the cardiac arrest team. In particular, there is a big emphasis on cardiac arrest prevention and the ABCDE approach to assess an acutely ill patient. For further information see www.resus.org.uk.

Care of the Critically Ill Surgical Patient (CCrISP™)
This 2.5-day course is designed to advance the practical, theoretical and personal skills necessary for the care of critically ill surgical patients. It is aimed at surgeons and those dealing with surgical patients who are completing basic surgical training. All participants on the course should have completed at least 1 year of basic surgical training (not including house jobs), should have commenced 6 months general surgery and should ideally have completed an ATLS course, although this is not a prerequisite.

START Surgery
The Systematic Training in Acute Illness Recognition and Treatment for Surgery (START Surgery) course is designed for surgical foundation trainees. It is designed to advance the practical, theoretical and personal skills necessary for the care of critically ill surgical patients. For further information see www.rcseng.ac.uk.

CONCLUSION
Critically ill patients have a high morbidity and high mortality. Prognosis following an in-hospital cardiopulmonary arrest is poor. Prompt recognition and early appropriate management of critically ill patients are essential to prevent deterioration. Tack and trigger systems should be in place to identify at-risk patients and alert expert help. Healthcare staff should be appropriately trained.

REFERENCES
Adam, S. & Osborne, S. (2005) *Critical Care Nursing Science and Practice* 2nd edn. Oxford University Press, Oxford.
Baudouin, S. & Evans, T. (2002) Improving outcomes for severely ill medical patients. *Clinical Medicine* (March/April) Editorial.
Bellomo, R., Goldsmith, D., Shigehiko, U. *et al.* (2003) A prospective before and after trial of a medical emergency team. *Medical Journal of Australia* **179** (6), 283–287.
Bristow, P.J., Hillman, K.M., Chey, T. *et al.* (2000) Rates of in-hospital arrests, deaths and intensive care admissions: the effect of the medical emergency team. *Medical Journal of Australia* **173**, 236–240.
Buist, M., Jarmolowski, E., Burton, P. *et al.* (1999) Recognising clinical instability in hospital patients before cardiac arrest or unplanned admission to intensive care. *Medical Journal of Australia* **171**, 22–25.

Buist, M., Moore, G., Bernard, S. *et al.* (2002) Effects of a medical emergency team on reduction of incidence of and mortality from unexpected cardiac arrests in hospital: preliminary study. *British Medical Journal* **324**, 1–5.

Buist, M., Bernard, S., Nguyen, T.V. *et al.* (2004) Association between clinically abnormal observations and subsequent in-hospital mortality: a prospective study. *Resuscitation* **62**, 137–141.

Cutherbertson, B. (2003) Outreach critical care – cash for no questions? *British Journal of Anaesthesia* **90** (1), 5–6.

Department of Health (2000) *Comprehensive Critical Care.* Department of Health, London.

Dhond, G., Ridley, S. & Palmer, M. (1998) The impact of a high-dependency unit on the workload of an intensive care unit. *Anaesthesia* **53**, 841–847.

Edbrooke, D., Hibbert, C. & Corcoran, M. (1999) *Review for the NHS Executive of Adult Critical Care Services: an International Perspective.* Medical Economics and Research Centre, Sheffield.

Fieselmann, J.F., Hendryx, M.S., Helms, C.M. *et al.* (1993) Respiratory rate predicts cardiopulmonary arrest for internal medicine patients. *Journal of General Internal Medicine* **8**, 354–360.

Franklin, C. & Mathew, J. (1994) Developing strategies to prevent in-hospital cardiac arrest: analyzing responses of physicians and nurses in the hours before the event. *Critical Care Medicine* **22**, 244–247.

Goldhill, D. (2001) The critically ill: following your MEWS. *QJM* **94**, 507–510.

Goldhill, D. & McNarry, A. (2004) The longer patients are in hospital before intensive care admission the higher their mortality. *Intensive Care Medicine* **30**, 1908–1913.

Goldhill, D.R., Worthington, L., Mulcahy, A. *et al.* (1999) The patient-at-risk team: identifying and managing seriously ill patients. *Anaesthesia* **54**, 853–860.

Gwinnutt, C. (2006) *Clinical Anaesthesia* 2nd edn. Blackwell Publishing, Oxford.

Gwinnutt, C.L., Columb, M. & Harris, R. (2000) Outcome after cardiac arrest in adults in UK hospitals: effect of the 1997 guidelines. *Resuscitation* **47**, 125–135.

Hodgetts, T.J., Kenward, G., Vlackonikolis, I. *et al.* (2002) Incidence, location and reasons for avoidable in-hospital cardiac arrest in a district general hospital. *Resuscitation* **54**, 115–123.

Holder, P. & Cuthbertson, B. (2005) Critical care without the intensive care unit. *Clinical Medicine* **5**, 449–451.

Intensive Care Society (2002) *Evolution of intensive care in the UK.* Intensive Care Society, London.

Kause, J., Smith, G., Prytherch, D. *et al.* (2004) A comparison of antecedents to cardiac arrests, deaths and emergency intensive care admissions in Australia and New Zealand, and the United Kingdom – the ACADEMIA study. *Resuscitation* **62**, 275–282.

Kruger, P. & Longden, P. (1997) A study of a hospital staff's knowledge of pulse oximetry. *Anaesthesia and intensive care* **25**, 38–41.

Lee, A., Bishop, G., Hillman, K. & Daffurn, K. (1995) The Medical Emergency Team. *Anaesthesia and Intensive Care* **23**, 183–186.

McGloin, H., Adam, S.K. *et al.* (1999) Unexpected deaths and referrals to intensive care of patients on general wards. Are some cases potentially preventable? *Journal of the Royal College of Physicians* **33** (3), 255–259.

McQuillan, P., Pilkington, S., Allan, A. *et al.* (1998) Confidential enquiry into quality of care before admission to intensive care. *British Medical Journal* **316**, 1853–1858.

Meek, T. (2000) New house officers' knowledge of resuscitation, fluid balance and analgesia. *Anaesthesia* **55**, 1128–1129.

NCEPOD (2005) *An Acute Problem?* National Confidential Enquiry into Patient Outcome and Death, London.

Nolan, J., Deakin, C., Soar, J. *et al.* (2005) European Resuscitation Council Guidelines for Resuscitation 2005: Section 4. Adult advanced life support. *Resuscitation* **675S**, S39–S86.

Parr, M. (2004) Critical care outreach: some answers, more questions. *Intensive Care Medicine* **30**, 1261–1262.

Resuscitation Council (UK) (2006) *Advanced Life Support* 5th edn. Resuscitation Council UK, London.

Rich, K. (1999) In-hospital cardiac arrest: pre-event variables and nursing response. *Clinical Nurse Specialist* 147–153.

Schein, R.M.H., Hazday, N., Pena, M. *et al.* (1990) Clinical antecedents to in-hospital cardiac arrest. *Chest* **98**, 1388–1392.

Sharpley, J.T. & Holden, J.C. (2004) Introducing an early warning scoring system in a district general hospital. *Nursing in Critical Care* **9** (3), 98–103.

Smith, A.F. & Wood, J. (1998) Can some in-hospital cardio-respiratory arrests be prevented? *Resuscitation* **37**, 133–137.

Smith, G. & Poplett, N. (2002) Knowledge of aspects of acute care in trainee doctors. *Postgraduate Medical Journal* **78**, 335–338.

Subbe, C.P., Davies, R.G., Williams, E. *et al.* (2003) Effect of introducing the modified early warning score on clinical outcomes, cardio-pulmonary arrests and intensive care utilisation in acute medical admissions. *Anaesthesia* **58**, 775–803.

Young, M.P., Gooder, V.J., McBride, K. *et al.* (2003) Inpatient transfers to the Intensive Care Unit. *Journal of General Internal Medicine* **18**, 77–83.

Assessment of the Critically Ill Patient

2

INTRODUCTION

Cardiopulmonary arrests occurring in patients in unmonitored ward areas are usually neither sudden nor unpredictable and are rarely caused by primary cardiac disease (Nolan *et al*. 2005). These patients have often slowly and progressively deteriorated physiologically, involving hypoxia and hypotension, which has not been recognised by ward staff, or if it has, has been poorly treated (Kause *et al*. 2004). If adverse physiological signs, e.g. tachycardia, tachypnoea or hypotension, are identified early, and patients are effectively treated, cardiopulmonary arrest may then be prevented (Adam & Osborne 2005).

The Resuscitation Council (UK) has provided guidance on the assessment of the critically ill patient (Resuscitation Council UK 2006). Adapted from the ALERT course (Smith 2003), these guidelines follow a logical and systematic ABCDE approach.

The aim of this chapter is to understand the assessment of the critically ill patient.

LEARNING OBJECTIVES

At the end of the chapter the reader will be able to:

❏ outline the ABCDE approach
❏ outline the initial approach to the patient
❏ describe the assessment of the airway
❏ describe the assessment of breathing
❏ outline the assessment of circulation
❏ describe the assessment of disability
❏ outline the importance of exposure

ABCDE APPROACH

The ABCDE approach can be used when assessing and treating all critically ill patients. The guiding principles are as follows:

- Follow a systematic approach, based on **A**irway, **B**reathing, **C**irculation, **D**isability and **E**xposure (ABCDE) to assess and treat the critically ill patient.
- Undertake a complete initial assessment; re-assess regularly.
- Always treat life-threatening problems first, before proceeding to the next part of the assessment.
- Always evaluate the effects of treatment and/or other interventions.
- Recognise the circumstances when additional help is required; request it early and utilise all members of the multi-disciplinary team. This will enable assessment, instigating monitoring, intravenous (IV) access etc. to be undertaken simultaneously.
- Ensure effective communication. Call for help early.

(Resuscitation Council UK 2006)

The ABCDE approach can be used by all healthcare practitioners, irrespective of their training, experience and expertise in clinical assessment and treatment: clinical skills and knowledge will determine what aspects of the assessment are undertaken (Resuscitation Council UK 2006).

> 'The underlying aim of the initial interventions should be seen as a "holding measure" to keep the patient alive, and produce some clinical improvement, in order that definitive treatment may be initiated' (Resuscitation Council UK 2005).

INITIAL APPROACH TO THE PATIENT

Ensure it is safe to approach the patient: check the environment and remove any hazards. Measures should also be taken to minimise the risk of cross infection (see box at end of chapter).

Ask the patient a simple question

Ask the patient a simple question, e.g. 'How are you, sir?' The patient's response or lack of response can provide valuable information. A normal verbal response implies that the patient has a patent airway, is breathing and has cerebral perfusion; if the patient can only speak in short sentences, he may have extreme respiratory distress and failure to respond is a clear indicator of serious illness (Resuscitation Council UK 2006). If there is an inappropriate response or no response, the patient may be critically ill.

If the patent is unconscious: summon help from colleagues immediately.

General appearance of the patient
Note the general appearance of the patient, e.g. whether he appears comfortable or distressed, content or concerned, and his colour.

Vital signs' monitoring
Equipment for vital signs' monitoring, e.g. pulse oximetry, electrocardiogram (ECG) monitoring and continuous non-invasive blood pressure monitoring, should be attached as soon as it is safely possible (Resuscitation Council UK 2006).

ASSESSMENT OF AIRWAY
If the patient is talking he will have a patent airway. In complete airway obstruction, there are no breath sounds at the mouth or nose. In partial obstruction, air entry is diminished and often noisy. The familiar look, listen and feel approach can detect if the airway is obstructed.

Look
Look for the signs of airway obstruction. Airway obstruction leads to paradoxical chest and abdominal movements ('see-saw' respirations) and the use of the accessory muscles of respiration. Central cyanosis is a late sign of airway obstruction.

Listen
Listen for signs of airway obstruction. Certain noises will assist in localising the level of the obstruction (Smith 2003):

- *Gurgling*: fluid in the mouth or upper airway.
- *Snoring*: tongue partially obstructing the pharynx.
- *Crowing*: laryngeal spasm.
- *Inspiratory stridor*: 'croaking respirations' indicating partial upper airway obstruction, e.g. foreign body, laryngeal oedema.
- *Expiratory wheeze*: noisy musical sound caused by turbulent flow of air through narrowed bronchi and bronchioles, more

pronounced on expiration; causes include asthma and chronic obstructive airways disorder.

Feel

Feel for signs of airway obstruction. Place your face or hand in front of the patient's mouth to determine whether there is movement of air.

Causes of airway obstruction

Causes of airway obstruction include:

- *Tongue* (this is the commonest cause of airway obstruction in a semi-conscious or unconscious patient; relaxation of the muscles supporting the tongue can result in it falling back and blocking the pharynx)
- *Vomit, blood and secretions*
- *Foreign body*
- *Tissue swelling* (causes include anaphylaxis, trauma or infection)
- *Laryngeal oedema* (due to burns, inflammation or allergy occurring at the level of the larynx)
- *Laryngeal spasm* (due to foreign body, airway stimulation or secretions/blood in the airway)
- *Tracheobronchial obstruction* (due to aspiration of gastric contents, secretions, pulmonary oedema fluid or bronchospasm)

(Smith 2003; Gwinnutt 2006)

Treatment of airway obstruction

Treat airway obstruction as a medical emergency and obtain expert help immediately; untreated, airway obstruction leads to a lowered PaO_2 and risks hypoxic damage to the brain, kidneys and heart, cardiac arrest, and even death (Resuscitation Council UK, 2006).

Once airway obstruction has been identified, treat appropriately. Simple methods, e.g. suction, lateral position, insertion of oropharyngeal airway, are often effective. Administer oxygen as appropriate.

Monitoring the patient's airway is described in more detail in Chapter 3.

ASSESSMENT OF BREATHING

The familiar look, listen and feel approach can be used to assess breathing, to detect signs of respiratory distress or inadequate ventilation (Smith 2003).

Look

Look for the general signs of respiratory distress: tachypnoea, sweating, central cyanosis, use of the accessory muscles of respiration, abdominal breathing (Resuscitation Council UK 2006).

Calculate the respiratory rate over 1 minute. The respiratory rate is the most useful sign that breathing is compromised (Smith 2003). The normal respiratory rate in adults is approximately 12–20 per minute (Resuscitation Council UK 2006). Tachypnoea is usually one of the first indicators of respiratory distress (Smith 2003). If the respiratory rate is high or increasing, this could indicate that the patient is ill and may suddenly deteriorate (Resuscitation Council UK 2006).

Bradypnoea is an ominous sign and possible causes include drugs (e.g. opiates), fatigue, hypothermia, head injury and central nervous system (CNS) depression. Sudden bradypnoea in a patient with respiratory distress could quickly be followed by respiratory arrest.

Assess the depth of breathing. Ascertain whether chest movement is equal on both sides. Unilateral movement of the chest suggests unilateral disease, e.g. pneumothorax, pneumonia or pleural effusion (Smith 2003). Kussmaul's breathing (air hunger) is characterised by deep rapid respirations due to stimulation of the respiratory centre by metabolic acidosis, e.g. in ketoacidosis, chronic renal failure.

Assess the pattern (rhythm) of breathing. Cheyne-Stokes breathing pattern (periods of apnoea alternating with periods of hyperpnoea) can be associated with brainstem ischaemia, cerebral injury and severe left ventricular failure (altered carbon dioxide sensitivity of the respiratory centre) (Ford *et al.* 2005).

Note the presence of any chest deformity because this could increase the risk of deterioration in the patient's ability to breathe normally (Resuscitation Council UK 2006). If the patient has a chest drain, check it is patent and functioning effectively. The presence of abdominal distension could limit diaphragmatic movement, thereby exacerbating respiratory distress.

Document the inspired oxygen concentration (percentage) being administered to the patient and the oxygen saturation (SaO_2) reading of the pulse oximeter (normally 97–100%). The pulse oximeter does not detect hypercapnia and, if the patient is receiving oxygen therapy, the SaO_2 may be normal in the presence of a very high $PaCO_2$ (Resuscitation Council UK 2006).

Listen

Listen to the patient's breath sounds a short distance from his face. Normal breathing is quiet. Rattling airway noises indicate the presence of airway secretions, usually either because the patient is unable to cough sufficiently or is unable to take a deep breath in (Smith 2003). Stridor or wheeze suggests partial, but significant, airway obstruction (see above).

If you are able, auscultate the chest: the depth of breathing and the equality of breath sounds on both sides of the chest should be evaluated. Any additional sounds, e.g. crackles, wheeze and pleural rubs, should be noted. Bronchial breathing indicates lung consolidation; absent or reduced sounds suggest a pneumothorax or pleural fluid (Smith 2003).

Feel

Perform chest percussion. Causes of different percussion notes include:

- *resonant*: air-filled lung
- *dull*: liver, spleen, heart, lung consolidation/collapse
- *stoney dull*: pleural effusion/thickening
- *hyper-resonant*: pneumothorax, emphysema
- *tympanitic*: gas-filled viscus

(Ford *et al*. 2005)

Check the position of the trachea. Place the tip of the index finger into the suprasternal notch, let it slip either side of the trachea and determine whether it fits more easily into one or other side of the trachea (Ford *et al*. 2005). Deviation of the trachea to one side indicates mediastinal shift (e.g. pneumothorax, lung fibrosis or pleural fluid).

Palpate the chest wall to detect surgical emphysema or crepitus (suggesting a pneumothorax *until* proven otherwise) (Smith 2003).

Efficacy of breathing, work of breathing and adequacy of ventilation

- *Efficacy of breathing* can be assessed by air entry, chest movement, pulse oximetry, arterial blood gas analysis and capnography.
- *Work of breathing* can be assessed by respiratory rate and accessory muscle use, e.g. neck and abdominal muscles.
- *Adequacy of ventilation* can be assessed by heart rate, skin colour and mental status.

Causes of compromised breathing

Causes of compromised breathing include:

- respiratory illness, e.g. asthma, chronic obstructive pulmonary disease (COPD), pneumonia
- lung pathology, e.g. pneumothorax
- pulmonary embolism
- pulmonary oedema
- central nervous system depression
- drug-induced respiratory depression

Treatment of compromised breathing

If the patient's breathing is compromised, position him appropriately (usually upright), administer oxygen and if possible treat the underlying cause. Expert help should be summoned. Assisted ventilation may be required. During the initial assessment of breathing, it is essential to diagnose and effectively treat immediately life-threatening conditions, e.g. acute severe asthma, pulmonary oedema, tension pneumothorax, massive haemothorax (Resuscitation Council UK 2006).

Assessment and monitoring of the patient's breathing is discussed in more detail in Chapter 3.

ASSESSMENT OF CIRCULATION

In most medical and surgical emergencies, if shock is present, treat for hypovolaemic shock until proven otherwise (Smith 2003).

Administer IV fluid to all patients who have tachycardia and cool peripheries, unless the cause of the circulatory shock is obviously cardiac (cardiogenic shock) (Resuscitation Council UK 2006). In surgical patients, haemorrhage should be rapidly excluded. The familiar look, listen and feel approach can be used for the assessment of circulation.

Look

Look at the colour of the hands and fingers. Signs of cardiovascular compromise include cool and pale peripheries.

Measure the capillary refill time (CRT). A prolonged CRT (>2 seconds) could indicate poor peripheral perfusion, though other factors, e.g. cool ambient temperature, poor lighting and old age, can also do this (Resuscitation Council UK 2006). Look for other signs of a poor cardiac output, e.g. reduced conscious level and, if the patient has a urinary catheter, oliguria (urine volume <0.5 ml/kg/hour) (Smith 2003).

Examine the patient for signs of external haemorrhage from wounds or drains or evidence of internal haemorrhage. Concealed blood loss can be significant, even if drains are empty (Smith 2003).

Listen

Measure the patient's blood pressure. A low systolic blood pressure suggests shock. However, even in shock, the blood pressure can still be normal, as compensatory mechanisms increase peripheral resistance in response to reduced cardiac output (Smith 2003). A low diastolic blood pressure suggests arterial vasodilatation (e.g. anaphylaxis or sepsis). A narrowed pulse pressure, i.e. the difference between systolic and diastolic pressures (normal pulse pressure is 35–45 mmHg), suggests arterial vasoconstriction (e.g. cardiogenic shock or hypovolaemia) (Resuscitation Council UK 2006).

Auscultate the heart. Although abnormalities of the heart valves can be detected, auscultation of the heart is rarely helpful in the initial assessment (Smith 2003).

Feel

Assess the skin temperature of the patient's limbs to determine whether they are warm or cool, the latter suggesting poor peripheral perfusion. Palpate peripheral and central pulses. Assess for presence, rate, quality, regularity and equality (Smith 2003). A thready pulse suggests a poor cardiac output, whilst a bounding pulse may indicate sepsis (Resuscitation Council UK 2006). Assess the state of the veins: if hypovolaemia is present the veins could be under-filled or collapsed (Smith 2003).

Causes of circulatory compromise

Causes of circulatory problems include:

- acute coronary syndromes
- cardiac arrhythmias
- shock, e.g. hypovolaemia, septic and anaphylactic shock
- heart failure
- pulmonary embolism

Treatment of circulatory compromise

The specific treatment required for circulatory compromise will depend on the cause; fluid replacement, haemorrhage control and restoration of tissue perfusion will usually be necessary (Resuscitation Council UK 2006).

The immediate treatment for a patient with an acute coronary syndrome includes oxygen, aspirin 300 mg, sublingual glyceryl trinitrate and morphine (diamorphine); reperfusion therapy will need to be considered (Resuscitation Council UK 2006). If shock is present, a large-bore cannula (12–14 gauge) should be inserted and an IV fluid challenge will usually be required.

Assessment and monitoring of the patient's circulation are discussed in more detail in Chapters 4 and 5.

ASSESSMENT OF DISABILITY

Assessment of disability involves evaluating central nervous system function. Undertake a rapid assessment of the patient's level of consciousness using the AVPU method (Fig. 1.4) (the Glasgow coma scale can also be used). Causes of altered conscious level include hypoxia, hypercapnia, cerebral hypoperfusion, the recent administration of sedatives/analgesic medications and hypoglycaemia (Resuscitation Council UK 2006). Therefore:

- Review ABC to exclude hypoxaemia and hypotension.
- Check the patient's drug chart for reversible drug-induced causes of altered conscious level.
- Undertake bedside glucose measurement to exclude hypoglycaemia.
- Examine the pupils (size, equality and reaction to light).

(Resuscitation Council UK 2006)

Causes of altered conscious level

Causes of altered conscious level include:

- severe hypoxia
- poor cerebral perfusion
- drugs, e.g. sedatives, opiates
- cerebral pathology
- hypercapnia
- hypoglycaemia
- alcohol

Treatment of altered conscious level

The first priority is to assess ABC: exclude or treat hypoxia and hypotension (Resuscitation Council UK 2006). If drug-induced altered conscious level is suspected and the effects are reversible, administer an antidote, e.g. naloxone for opiate toxicity. Administer glucose if the patient is hypoglycaemic.

Assessment and monitoring of the patient's conscious level is discussed in more detail in Chapter 6.

EXPOSURE

Full exposure of the patient may be necessary in order to undertake a thorough examination and ensure important details are not overlooked (Smith 2003). In particular, the examination should concentrate on the part of the body which is most likely to be contributing to the patient's ill status, e.g. in suspected anaphylaxis, examine the skin for urticaria. The patient's dignity should be respected and heat loss minimised.

In addition:

- Undertake a full clinical history.
- Review the patient's case notes, observations chart and medications chart.

- Study the recorded vital signs: trends are more significant than one-off recordings.
- Ensure that prescribed medications are being administered.
- Review the results of laboratory, ECG and radiological investigations.
- Consider the level of care the patient requires (e.g. ward, HDU, ICU).
- Record in the patient's case notes details of assessment, treatment and response to treatment.

(Resuscitation Council UK 2006)

Minimising the risk of cross infection

Measures to minimise the risk of cross infection should be taken. It is estimated that 5000 deaths per year are directly associated with hospital-acquired infection (HAI) and in 15000 deaths per year it is a contributory factor (Plowman *et al.* 1997). The principal route of HAI is via the hands (Casewell & Phillips 1977; Elliott 1992; Bursey *et al.* 2001). Effective hand hygiene is recognised as the most effective intervention to prevent cross infection (Larson 1999; Bissett 2003; NICE 2003) and is the simplest (Voss & Widmer 1997).

The National Institute for Clinical Excellence (NICE) (2003) has issued guidance governing the principles of good practice relating to hand washing:

- Hands must be decontaminated immediately before each patient and every episode of direct patient contact or care after any activity or contact that could potentially result in hands becoming decontaminated.
- Hands that are visibly soiled, or potentially grossly contaminated with dirt or organic material, must be washed with liquid soap and water.
- Hands must be decontaminated, preferably with an alcohol-based handrub unless hands are visibly soiled, between caring for different patients and between different care activities for the same patient.
- Before regular hand decontamination begins, all wrist and ideally hand jewellery should be removed. Cuts and abrasions must be covered with waterproof dressings. Fingernails should be kept short, clean and free from nail polish.

Continued

- An effective handwashing technique involves three stages: preparation, washing and rinsing, and drying. Preparation requires wetting hands under tepid running water before applying liquid soap or an antimicrobial preparation. The handwash solution must come into contact with all surfaces of the hand. The hands must be rubbed together vigorously for a minimum of 10–15 seconds, paying particular attention to the tips of the fingers, the thumbs and the areas between the fingers. Hands should be rinsed thoroughly before drying with good-quality paper towels.
- When decontaminating hands using an alcohol handrub, hands should be free from dirt and organic material. The handrub solution must come into contact with all surfaces of the hand. The hands must be rubbed together, paying particular attention to the tips of the fingers, the thumbs and the areas between the fingers, until the solution has evaporated and the hands are dry.
- An emollient hand cream should be applied regularly to protect skin from the drying effects of regular hand decontamination. If a particular soap, antimicrobial hand wash or alcohol product causes skin irritation an occupational health team should be consulted.

For hygienic hand disinfection, an antiseptic solution will need to be used, e.g. chlorhexidine (Bursey *et al.* 2001). This category of handwashing should be used during an infection outbreak, prior to aseptic techniques and when the hands have been contaminated with body fluids (Kerr 1998). It is also recommended to use hygienic hand disinfection in particularly vulnerable patients, e.g. those who are immunodepressed, ICU patients and in newborn babies (Horton & Parker 1997).

Universal precautions to blood and bodily fluids

Blood is the single most important source of the transmission of human immunodeficiency virus (HIV) and hepatitis B virus (Jevon 2001). Universal precautions should apply to blood, semen, vaginal secretions and cerebrospinal, synovial, pleural, peritoneal, pericardial and amniotic fluids and any body fluid containing visible blood. Disposable gloves should be worn.

Sharps

Particular care should be taken with sharps as both HIV and the hepatitis B virus have been contracted by healthcare workers following needle-stick injuries.

CONCLUSION

Most cardiopulmonary arrests occurring in hospital are predictable. Recognition and the effective treatment of critically ill patients is paramount. The ABCDE approach of assessing the critically ill patient has been described and the importance of calling for help early has been emphasised.

REFERENCES

Adam, S. & Osborne, S. (2005) *Critical Care Nursing Science and Practice* 2nd edn. Oxford University Press, Oxford.

Bissett, L. (2003) Interpretation of terms used to describe handwashing activities. *British Journal of Nursing* **12** (9), 536–542.

Bursey, S., Hardy, C. & Gregson, R. (2001) Handwashing. *Professional Nurse* **16** (10), 1417–1416.

Casewell, M. & Phillips, I. (1977) Hands as route of transmission for *Klebsiella* species. *British Medical Journal* **2**, 1315–1317.

Elliott, P. (1992) Hand washing: a process of judgement and effective decision making. *Professional Nurse* **2**, 292–296.

Ford, M., Hennessey, I. & Japp, A. (2005) *Introduction to clinical examination.* Elsevier, Oxford.

Gwinnutt, C. (2006) *Clinical Anaesthesia* 2nd edn. Blackwell Publishing, Oxford.

Horton, R. & Parker, L. (1997) *Informed Infection Control Practice.* Churchill Livingstone, London.

Jevon, P. (2001) *Advanced Cardiac Life Support.* Butterworth Heinemann, Oxford.

Kause, J., Smith, G., Prytherch, D. *et al.* (2004) A comparison of antecedents to cardiac arrests, deaths and emergency intensive care admissions in Australia and New Zealand, and the United Kingdom – the ACADEMIA study. *Resuscitation* **62**, 275–282.

Kerr, J. (1998) Handwashing. *Nursing Standard* **12** (51), 35–42.

Larson, E. (1999) Skin hygiene and infection prevention: more of the same or different approaches? *Clinical Infectious Diseases* **29**, 1287–1294.

National Institute for Clinical Excellence (2003) *Head Injury, Triage, Assessment, Investigation and Early Management of Head Injury in Infants, Children and Adults.* NICE, London.

Plowman, R., Graves, N. & Roberts, J. (1997) *Hospital Acquired Infection.* Office of Health Economics, London.

Resuscitation Council (UK) (2006) *Advanced Life Support* 5th edn. Resuscitation Council UK, London.

Smith, G. (2003) *ALERT Acute Life-Threatening Events Recognition and Treatment* 2nd edn. University of Portsmouth, Portsmouth.

Voss, A. & Widmer, A. (1997) No time for hand-washing? Handwashing vs alcohol rubs: can we afford 100% compliance? *Infection Control and Hospital Epidemiology* **18**, 205–208.

3 | Monitoring Respiratory Function

INTRODUCTION

Early recognition of respiratory dysfunction and the institution of appropriate measures are vital to support gas exchange and prevent cellular oxygen debt, anaerobic metabolism and varying degrees of tissue and organ damage (Smyth 2005).

Respiratory function requires careful and close monitoring to ensure the most appropriate treatment is administered and any response to it is accurately evaluated. Table 3.1 shows the basic definitions of respiratory terminology and Table 3.2 some of the most common causes of dyspnoea (breathing difficulty).

In particular it is important to be able to recognise when the patient's respiratory status is compromised. The familiar *look*, *listen* and *feel* approach can be used to evaluate the efficacy of breathing, work of breathing and adequacy of ventilation. The patient's general appearance, history and presenting symptoms together with the characteristics of the dyspnoea are also important. Peak flow measurements, pulse oximetry and blood gas analysis are also helpful in monitoring respiratory function.

The aim of this chapter is to understand the principles of monitoring respiratory function.

LEARNING OBJECTIVES

At the end of the chapter the reader will be able to:

❏ describe how to assess the *efficacy of breathing, work of breathing* and *adequacy of ventilation*
❏ discuss the importance of a *comprehensive assessment* of the patient
❏ outline important *associated features of dyspnoea*
❏ describe how to undertake *peak expiratory flow rate measurements*
❏ discuss the principles of *pulse oximetry*

❏ discuss the principles of *arterial blood gas analysis*
❏ discuss the principles of *capnography*
❏ discuss the monitoring priorities of a *ventilated patient*
❏ discuss the monitoring priorities of a patient with a *temporary tracheostomy*
❏ outline the monitoring priorities of a patient with a *chest drain*

Table 3.1 Definitions of respiratory terminology.

Term	Definition
Dyspnoea	Difficulty in breathing
Orthopnoea	Dyspnoea necessitating an upright, sitting position for its relief
Tachypnoea	Abnormally rapid rate of breathing (>20 per minute) (Torrance & Elley 1997)
Bradypnoea	Abnormally slow rate of breathing (<12 per minute) (Torrance & Elley 1997)
Hypoxia	Inadequate oxygen at cellular level
Hypoxaemia	Low oxygen levels in the blood
Anoxia	Lack of oxygen, local or systemic

ASSESSMENT OF THE EFFICACY OF BREATHING, WORK OF BREATHING AND ADEQUACY OF VENTILATION

Efficacy of breathing

The efficacy of breathing can be assessed by the following:

• *Air entry*: look, listen and feel for signs of breathing. If able, auscultate the chest to determine the amount of air being inspired/expired in the apices and bases. A silent chest is an ominous sign.
• *Chest movement*: is chest movement equal, bilateral and symmetrical? The depth of inspiration should be noted (Simpson 2006).

Table 3.2 Causes of dyspnoea (not exhaustive).

Cause	Examples
Respiratory	Asthma, chronic obstructive pulmonary disease (COPD), pneumonia, tuberculosis, pleural effusion, pneumothorax, carcinoma of the lung, pulmonary embolism, mechanical (e.g. fractured ribs – flail segment)
Cardiac	Left ventricular failure and pulmonary oedema, congestive cardiac failure
CNS	Head injury, raised intracranial pressure, drugs (e.g. opiates); aggravating factors, e.g. exercise, cold air, smoking, coughing
Neuromuscular	Guillain–Barre syndrome, myasthenia gravis, muscular dystrophies
Diabetes	Hyperventilation in ketoacidosis
Pregnancy	
Obesity	
Anaemia	

Adapted from Jevon & Ewens 2001.

- *Pulse oximetry*: continuous peripheral oxygen saturation monitoring.
- *Arterial blood gas analysis*: the definitive method to assess the effectiveness of ventilation.

Work of breathing

Healthy spontaneous breathing is quiet and accomplished with minimal effort (Jevon & Ewens 2001). Signs of increased work of breathing include a rise in *respiratory rate, noisy respirations* and *use of accessory muscles.*

Respiratory rate

Changes to the rate and depth of respiration can be indicative of many conditions (Trim 2005). A rise in the respiratory rate has been recognised as one of the first indicators of deterioration and antecedent to adverse events (Schein *et al.* 1990; Buist *et al.* 1999; Goldhill *et al.* 1999; McGloin *et al.* 1999; Rich, 1999; Crispin & Daffurn 2000). The normal respiratory rate in adults is approximately 12 breaths per minute; tachypnoea (>12 breaths per minute, Trim 2005) is usually one of the first indications of respiratory distress (Resuscitation Council UK 2006). Respiratory dysfunction prior to an adverse event is associated with an increased mortality (Considine 2005). Bradypnoea (<10 breaths per minute, Simpson 2006) may be an ominous sign and possible causes include drugs, e.g. opiates, fatigue, hypothermia and CNS depression. The following disturbed breathing patterns are also significant:

- *Kussmaul's breathing (air hunger)*: deep rapid respirations due to stimulation of the respiratory centre by metabolic acidosis, e.g. in ketoacidosis or chronic renal failure.
- *Cheyne-Stokes breathing pattern*: periods of apnoea alternating with periods of hyperpnoea; causes include left ventricular failure, renal failure, increased intracranial pressure (ICP), drug overdose (Simpson 2006) and cerebral injury; usually seen in the end stages of life.
- *Hyperventilation*: often associated with anxiety states.

Noisy respirations
The following symptoms are also indicative of breathing difficulty and can be heard without the aid of a stethoscope:

- *Stridor*: 'croaking' respiration which is louder during inspiration; caused by laryngeal or tracheal obstruction, e.g. foreign body, laryngeal oedema or laryngeal tumour.
- *Wheeze*: noisy musical sound caused by turbulent flow of air through narrowed bronchi and bronchioles, more pronounced on expiration; causes include asthma and chronic obstructive pulmonary disease (COPD).
- *'Rattly' chest*: e.g. chest infection, pulmonary oedema and sputum retention.
- *Gurgling*: caused by fluid in the upper airway.
- *Snoring*: snoring sounds may be associated with the tongue blocking the airway in an unconscious patient.

(Jevon & Ewens 2001)

Accessory muscle use
The use of accessory muscles is a further indication of breathing difficulty. However, in older people abdominal breathing is

considered normal but the use of neck and upper chest muscles as abnormal in all adults (Simpson 2006).

Adequacy of ventilation

The assessment of heart rate, skin colour and the patient's mental status can help provide an indication of the adequacy of ventilation. Hypoxaemia can affect the following:

- *Heart rate*: initially tachycardia (a non-specific sign), but severe hypoxaemia can cause bradycardia.
- *Skin colour*: initially pallor, hypoxia causes catecholamine release and vasoconstriction; central cyanosis is a late and often pre-terminal sign of hypoxaemia (if the patient is anaemic, severe hypoxaemia may not cause cyanosis).*
- *Mental status*: agitation (may be an early sign), drowsiness, confusion and impaired consciousness.

(Jevon & Ewens 2001)

*N.B. If the patient has chronic obstructive pulmonary disorder (COPD) or congenital heart disease, cyanosis may be 'constant'.

COMPREHENSIVE ASSESSMENT OF THE PATIENT

The following matters should all be investigated and taken into account to arrive at a comprehensive assessment of the patient's condition.

Severity

It is important to establish what is normal for the patient and the effect of the breathlessness on the patient (Jevon & Ewens 2001). Can the patient talk with ease? How far can the patient walk without having to stop? Can the patient climb the stairs? Is the patient orthopnoeic? If so how many pillows does the patient sleep with? Does breathlessness affect the patient's daily activities or job? Does the patient require oxygen at home?

Timing

Severe asthma and left ventricular failure are more common at night. Occupation-related asthma is worse when the patient is at work and improves when the patient is at home (Jevon & Ewens 2001). Bronchitis is more common in the winter months.

Finger clubbing

Finger clubbing can indicate pulmonary or cardiovascular disease; clinical features often include loss of nailbed angle, an increased curvature of the nail and swelling of the terminal part of the digit, this is usually as a result of chronic hypoxaemia (Simpson 2006).

Shape of the chest

The normal chest is bilaterally symmetrical, though it can be distorted by disease of the ribs or spinal vertebrae as well as by underlying lung disease. In kyphosis (forward bending) or scoliosis (lateral bending) of the vertebral column, lung movement can be severely restricted. A barrel chest is sometimes associated with chronic bronchitis and emphysema (Jevon & Ewens 2001).

Chest percussion

Percussion of the chest wall causes the chest wall and underlying tissues to move (Simpson 2006). As a result audible sounds and palpable vibrations are felt. Percussion is performed by placing one hand on the chest with fingers separated and the other hand is used as a hammer to tap the interphalangeal joint, moving down the chest at 3–4 cm intervals (Simpson 2006). Comparison should be made between the left and right sides of the chest.

Hyper-resonance (loud sound) to percussion is caused by an increase in air in the chest, e.g. emphysema, pneumothorax. Dense sound to percussion can be caused by thickening of the chest wall, lung consolidation or pleural effusion.

Auscultation of the chest

Normal breath sounds should be bilateral and audible in all lung zones (Bennett 2003). Diminished breath sounds can be caused by poor ventilation, e.g. airway obstruction, respiratory depression, or by increased separation of the stethoscope from the bronchial tree, e.g. obesity, pleural effusion, pneumothorax, bronchial tumour. Fine late inspiratory crackles may be heard, e.g. pulmonary oedema; coarse early inspiratory crackles are heard in bronchitis and bronchiectasis (Simpson 2006); a coarse rubbing sound indicates pleural inflammation.

Medications

Medications the patient is currently taking may be significant. For instance, beta blockers can exacerbate asthma and left ventricular failure.

Halitosis

This may indicate poor oral hygiene or could be a sign of an infection of the upper respiratory tract.

Patient's position and emotional state

Does the patient need to sit in a particular position, e.g. supported by a bed-table to facilitate breathing? Is the patient orthopnoeic? A breathless patient will be anxious.

Past medical history and family medical history

All previous illnesses, operations, hospital admissions and investigations, particularly those that are respiratory related, e.g. COPD, should be noted (Booker 2004). Has the patient been prescribed any respiratory related medication, e.g. inhalers or oxygen? If so the frequency and effectiveness of its use should be noted. Any respiratory disease in the patient's family should be noted.

Occupational and social history

When assessing respiratory disease, both past and present occupations together with any exposure to dust, asbestos, coal or animals could be significant. Smoking history, past and present consumption, should be noted, together with any exposure to infection, e.g. tuberculosis. The type of living accommodation may be significant, e.g. stairs, damp environment, lack of a working lift in a block of flats.

Patient's age

Certain respiratory diseases are more likely to occur at particular times of life: <30 years – asthma, pneumothorax, cystic fibrosis, congenital heart disease; >50 years – chronic bronchitis, chronic obstructive pulmonary disease (COPD), carcinoma of the lung, pneumoconiosis, ischaemic heart disease.

Recent travel

Patients who have recently arrived from the Asian subcontinent may have been exposed to tuberculosis or recently identified viruses such as avian influenza.

Allergies

Any allergies should be recorded in both the patient's medical and nursing notes and on the prescription administration chart. Dependent upon individual hospital policy the patient may be required to wear a red armband in addition to the above precautions.

ASSOCIATED SYMPTOMS OF DYSPNOEA

Chest pain

Respiratory-related chest pain or pleuritic pain is usually sharp in nature and aggravated by deep breathing or coughing. It is often localised to one particular area (Jevon & Ewens 2001). Stabbing sudden-onset pleuritic pain may indicate a pneumothorax or a pulmonary embolus whereas a dull generalised pain may indicate a pneumonia (Booker 2004).

Cough

A cough is a common respiratory symptom. It occurs when deep inspiration is followed by an explosive expiration. A cough that is worse at night is suggestive of asthma or heart failure, while a cough that is worse after eating is suggestive of oesophageal reflux. The timing and duration of the cough is important:

- *sudden cough*: may be due to a foreign body
- *recent cough*: may be due to a chest infection
- *chronic cough associated with a wheeze*: may be due to asthma
- *irritating chronic dry cough*: may be due to oesophageal reflux
- *chronic cough with production of large volumes of purulent sputum*: may be due to bronchiectasis
- *change in the character of a chronic cough*: may be due to a serious underlying pathology, e.g. carcinoma of the lung

(Jevon & Ewens 2001)

Sputum

Sputum is a key clinical feature of respiratory disease and can provide valuable information for the assessment of a breathless patient, including evaluation of care (Law 2000). If sputum is produced, its colour and consistency should be noted:

- *white mucoid sputum*: seen in asthma and chronic bronchitis
- *purulent green or yellow sputum*: may indicate respiratory infection
- *blood present*: may indicate carcinoma of the lung, pulmonary embolism (Brewis 1996), recent upper airway trauma or coagulation disorder
- *frothy white or pink sputum*: seen in pulmonary oedema
- *thick, viscid sputum*: feature of severe or life-threatening asthma (Bennett 2003)
- *thin, watery sputum*: associated with acute pulmonary oedema (Bennett 2003)
- *foul smelling sputum*: indication of respiratory tract infection
- *black specks*: common causes include smoke inhalation and coal dust

The patient's history is important when determining the significance of sputum production at a particular time of day, e.g. chronic expectoration in the morning over a number of years may be suggestive of smoking-induced bronchitis while variable morning or nocturnal expectoration may be suggestive of asthma (Law 2000).

Important coexisting clinical features

A number of important coexisting clinical features may be associated with respiratory problems, including:

- *fever*: respiratory infection
- *poor appetite and weight loss*: carcinoma of the lung, chronic infection
- *swollen and painful calf*: deep vein thrombosis and pulmonary embolism
- *ankle swelling*: congestive cardiac failure, deep vein thrombosis
- *palpitations*: cardiac arrhythmias

(Jevon & Ewens 2001)

MEASUREMENT OF PEAK EXPIRATORY FLOW RATE

Peak expiratory flow rate (PEF) or peak flow is the maximum flow rate, in litres per minute, attained on forced expiration from a position of full inspiration (Bennett 2003). It is a simple test to ascertain the severity of a patient's asthma and can provide the practitioner with a guide to the level of resistance within the bronchioles. This resistance can be caused by inflammation and/ or bronchospasm. Peak flow is not a measure of fitness or the strength of the patient's chest muscles.

Indications

Recordings should be undertaken four times a day, both before and after the administration of bronchodilators (Ross-Plummer 2000; Booker 2004). The results are crucial to the patient's treatment and are an aid to asthma diagnosis (Miller 2005), an indicator of how well the patient's asthma is responding to treatment and an aid to measuring the recovery from an asthma attack (Booker 2004; Miller 2005).

Normal range for peak expiratory flow rate measurement

The normal range for peak flow recordings is influenced by age, sex and height (Simpson 2006). Peak flow readings are usually higher in men than in women and the best peak flow usually occurs between the ages of 30 and 40 years (Partridge 1997). In addition it varies throughout the day; it is often higher in the evenings than in the mornings. It is therefore important to record peak flows at both these times.

Procedure

1. Explain the procedure to the patient.
2. Assemble the necessary equipment – mini-Wright flow meter, clean mouth piece, observation chart. Ensure the flow meter is set at zero.
3. If possible stand the patient up.
4. Ask the patient to take a deep breath in and place the peak flow meter in the mouth, holding it horizontally and closing the lips.
5. Ask the patient to breathe out as hard and as fast as possible.

6. Note the recording on the flow meter and then return it to zero.
7. Ask the patient to repeat the procedure twice.
8. Record the best of the three recordings.

(Adapted from Jevon *et al.* 2000)

PULSE OXIMETRY

Pulse oximetry is widely regarded as one of the greatest advances in clinical monitoring (Giuliano & Higgins 2005) since the invention of the ECG (Fox 2002) and is an essential monitoring and diagnostic tool both in critical care and ward areas (Mathews 2005). It is a simple, non-invasive bedside method of measuring arterial oxygen saturation (Leach, 2004; Higgins 2005) expressed as SpO_2 (Welch 2005). Pulse oximetry was developed in the 1980s; before this time oxygenation assessment was reliant on subjective and unreliable physical assessment of the skin for cyanosis (Giuliano & Higgins 2005) which when present is an indicator of advanced hypoxaemia (Giuliano 2006).

Pulse oximetry only measures the extent to which haemoglobin is saturated with oxygen and does not provide information on oxygen delivery to the tissues or ventilatory function (Higgins 2005). Nevertheless, it is an invaluable monitoring tool in a variety of clinical settings, as long as its uses and limitations are fully understood (Jevon & Ewens 2000; Giuliano 2006).

Role of pulse oximetry

Hypoxaemia is common in all aspects of medical practice and without appropriate treatment will lead to cellular death and organ dysfunction.

Cyanosis is a late sign of hypoxaemia and the oxygen saturation must decrease to 80–85% before any changes in skin colour become apparent (Giuliano & Higgins 2005). In addition, manifestations of hypoxaemia, including restlessness, confusion, agitation, cyanosis, combative behaviour and tachycardia (McEnroe Ayres & Stucky Lappin 2004), may be missed or wrongly interpreted (Technology Subcommittee of the Working Group on Critical Care 1992).

Pulse oximetry, the fifth vital sign (Welch 2005), will immediately alert the practitioner to a fall in arterial oxygen saturations and the development of hypoxaemia, prior to visual recognition of cyanosis. In clinical practice an oxygen saturation of less than 90% is of concern.

> The absence of cyanosis does not exclude severe hypoxaemia; it will not be present if the haemoglobin concentration is low or if there is poor perfusion of the capillaries (McEnroe Ayres & Stucky Lappin 2004).

The mechanics of pulse oximetry

Pulse oximetry (Fig. 3.1) is a differential measurement based on the spectrophotometric absorption method using the Beer-Lambert Law for optical absorption (Welch 2005).

The pulse oximeter probe consists of two light-emitting diodes (one red and one infrared) on one side of the probe. These transmit red and infrared light across the vascular bed, usually a finger tip or ear lobe, to a photodetector on the other side of the probe (Welch 2005). The ratio of absorption is relative to the concentration of oxygenated haemoglobin to deoxygenated haemoglobin (Welch 2005). The more oxygenated the blood is more red light

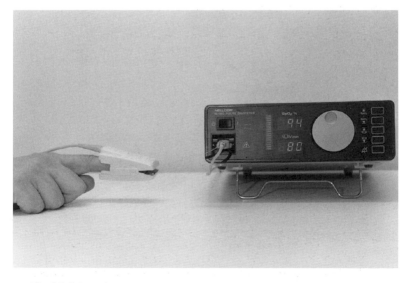

Fig. 3.1 Pulse oximeter.

passes through and less infrared light passes through (Giuliano 2006). By calculating the ratios of red to infrared light over time, oxygen saturation is calculated (Giuliano 2006).

Uses of pulse oximetry
Pulse oximetry is indicated in any clinical situation where hypoxaemia may occur (Hanning & Alexander-Williams 1995). It is used in a variety of clinical settings, including:

- theatres
- intensive care units
- emergency departments
- general wards
- endoscopy departments
- neonatal units
- patient transfer
- sleep studies
- primary care
- sleep study laboratories

Advantages of pulse oximetry
Pulse oximetry is an inexpensive, non-invasive and portable method of continuous measurement of arterial oxygen saturation which facilitates the early detection of hypoxaemia. It also provides information about the heart rate (Jevon & Ewens 2000; Welch 2005). Although analysis of arterial blood gases has been the gold standard for measuring arterial oxygen saturation, it is invasive, time-consuming, costly, involves repeated arterial blood sampling and only provides intermittent information (Jenson *et al.* 1998).

Normal values for oxygen saturation
The normal range for oxygen saturation measurements is >95% (Fox 2002; Booker 2004), though lower measurements may be 'normal' for some patients, e.g. COPD (Fox 2002; Bennett 2003).

Procedure for pulse oximetry
The following preliminary points should be observed:

- ensure the probe is clean

- wash and dry hands
- explain the procedure to the patient

Select an appropriate site with an adequate pulsating vascular bed. Sites include finger (most popular), ear lobe (less accurate, Jenson *et al.* 1998); toes can be used instead of fingers, but poor perfusion is more common (Hanning & Alexander-Williams 1995). Avoid application of the probe distal to blood pressure cuffs or arterial/venous lines. If the finger is used, remove any nail polish (Higgins 2005) (obtain patient's consent first). The probe should be secured, but without the use of restrictive tape. The following precautions must be taken during the procedure:

- Ensure that the trace is reliable and corresponds to pulse rate, i.e. oxygen saturation measurements are accurate (Fig. 3.2).
- Ensure the alarms on the pulse oximeter are set within locally agreed limits and according to the patient's condition.
- Regularly monitor the probe site for complications, e.g. burns and joint stiffness, and regularly vary the site.
- Regularly monitor the patient's vital signs.
- Document the readings and inform medical staff as appropriate.

(Adapted from Jevon & Ewens 2000)

Interpreting plethysmographic waveforms
The quality of the pulse and circulation at the point where SpO_2 is being measured is reflected in the plethysmographic waveform (Fig. 3.2); the strength of the pulse is proportional to the amplitude of the waveform (Place 2000).

Causes of inaccuracy
Inaccurate readings can be caused by any of the factors listed below:

- *Carbon monoxide poisoning*: false high readings (Mathews 2005).
- *Methaemoglobinaemia* (changes in the structure of iron in haemoglobin) and if present in high doses can give false high or low readings (Welch 2005).
- *Poor vascular perfusion*: pulse oximeter requires pulsatile blood flow to evaluate oxygen saturation.

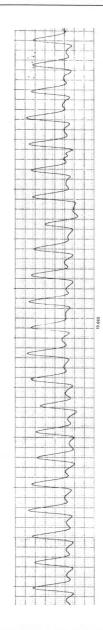

Fig. 3.2 SpO₂ waveform.

- *Venous pulsation*: e.g. tricuspid valve failure, securing the probe too tightly (Fox 2002; Welch 2005) heart failure, inflating blood pressure cuff distal to the probe, resulting in a false low reading.
- *Poor vascular perfusion*: e.g. in hypovolaemia, hypotension, septicaemia, hypothermia, cardiogenic shock or peripheral vascular disease, resulting in a false low reading.
- *Cardiac arrhythmias* such as atrial fibrillation can cause inadequate and irregular perfusion, resulting in a false low reading.
- *Factors that affect light absorption*: skin pigmentation, dried blood and dark nail polish (Welch 2005), and intravenous dyes, e.g. methylene blue (Fox 2002).
- *Bright external light*, particularly fluorescent lighting (Fox 2002; Gwinnutt 2006) can give a false high reading.
- *Anaemia* (Weston Smith *et al*. 1989; Severinghaus & Koh 1990).
- *Patient on supplementary oxygen* can mean that hypoxaemia will not be detected early (Hutton & Clutton-Brock 1993).
- *Oxygen saturations* ≤70% (Schnapp & Cohen 1990).
- *Patient movement*, e.g. shivering; though modern pulse oximeters can minimise the interference from patient movement (Gwinnutt 2006).

Limitations
Although pulse oximetry measures oxygen saturation and can detect hypoxaemia, it does not provide an indication of the adequacy of ventilation and carbon dioxide retention.

Davidson and Hosie (1993) reported a case of a post-operative patient who had a normal oxygen saturation (95%), but had abnormally high carbon dioxide levels causing a life-threatening respiratory acidosis. Failure to detect hypoventilation in such a patient is an example of a false sense of security generated by a single physiological variable being within safe limits (Hutton & Clutton-Brock 1993). If hypercapnia is suspected arterial blood gas analysis should be performed.

Troubleshooting
It is important to ensure a reliable trace at all times. If it is difficult to secure an acceptable trace:

- warm and rub the skin to improve circulation
- try a different probe site, e.g. ear lobe
- try a different probe/different pulse oximeter

Complications

Pulse oximetry is very safe; complications are uncommon and are rarely serious if they do occur (Richardson & Hale 1995). Nevertheless complications have been reported.

- *Ischaemic pressure necrosis* (Fox 2002): in the reported case the patient was septic, hypotensive and had pre-existing arterial disease. In addition an arterial line was *in situ* in the radial artery which may have further compromised the distal circulation.
- *Perioperative corneal abrasions*: resulting from patients rubbing their eyes with the index finger with probe and dressing attached (Brock-Utne *et al.* 1992).
- *Blister injuries at the probe site*: caused by a faulty probe cable; intermittent shortening resulting in excess electrical current supply to the light-emitting diode causing overheating.
- *Mechanical injury*: if the patient is unable to flex his finger; in unconscious or semiconscious patients the probe may inhibit

---

Best practice – pulse oximetry

Remove anything that could impair the translucence of the sensor site.

Position the probe without excessive force, i.e. avoid the use of adhesive tape.

Ensure an accurate trace is obtained.

Be aware of any past or presenting history which may give aberrant results.

Note any activity associated with a lower and higher SpO_2 reading.

Note the use of supplementary oxygen.

Compare results with previous readings and assess for any trends.

Always rely on clinical judgment rather than an SpO_2 reading in isolation.

Regularly monitor and alternate probe site.

Ensure the digit used is regularly flexed to avoid mechanical injury.

---

voluntary use of the finger, resulting in stiffness. Changing the probe site regularly is therefore advocated (Richardson & Hale 1995). This is potentially a problem for patients on ICUs where prolonged monitoring occurs.

ARTERIAL BLOOD GAS ANALYSIS

Arterial blood gas (ABG) analysis is one of the most common tests performed in the critically ill patient and has become an essential skill for all healthcare practitioners (Simpson 2004). It provides clinicians with valuable information about a patient's respiratory function and metabolic state (Shoulders-Odom 2000; Simpson 2004; Allen 2005) and as such forms an integral component of monitoring the critically ill patient. It is important to remember that, as with all assessment methods, ABG interpretation should not be taken in isolation (Simpson 2004).

Procedure for arterial blood sampling

There are two methods of arterial blood sampling, either from a one-off arterial puncture or 'stab' or from an arterial cannula. An arterial 'stab' is usually taken from the radial artery (Woodrow 2004), as it is most accessible. The femoral artery is also sometimes used.

The following procedure for arterial blood sampling is based on recommendations by Driscoll *et al.* (1997):

1. Ensure the three-way tap is closed to air. This is to prevent back-flow of blood and blood spillage.
2. Remove cap from three-way tap, clean the open port with an alcohol swab and connect a sterile 5 ml syringe.
3. Turn the tap to connect the artery to the syringe and aspirate 5 ml of blood. This will ensure that the sample of blood used for analysis is fresh and does not contain 'flush solution'. The tap is now 'off' to the flush solution.
4. Turn the tap off to the syringe; remove and discard the syringe.
5. Replace with a heparinised syringe and turn the tap to connect it to the artery.
6. Slowly aspirate the required amount of blood (Fig. 3.3) and then turn the tap off to the syringe. It is important to aspirate

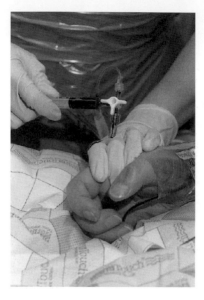

Fig. 3.3 Arterial blood sampling.

the blood slowly as this will help to prevent spasm in the vessel (Mallett & Dougherty 2000).

7. Remove the syringe and re-apply a new sterile cap, ensuring it is securely attached.
8. Flush the tubing and watch for return of reliable arterial trace on the monitor. Ensure that the infuser cuff is inflated to 300 mmHg (Mallett & Dougherty 2000).
9. Insert blood into the blood gas analyser according to manufacturer's recommendations being sure to include the patient's identification, temperature and any supplementary oxygen being administered (Fig. 3.4).
10. Document the results and inform medical staff if appropriate.

Indications for ABG analysis
Indications for ABG analysis include:

• respiratory compromise

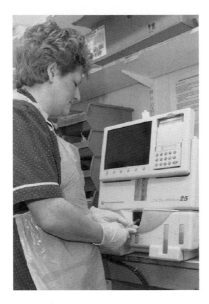

Fig. 3.4 Blood gas machine.

- post cardiopulmonary arrest
- metabolic conditions, e.g. diabetic ketoacidosis (DKA)
- sudden or unexplained deterioration
- evaluation of interventions, e.g. changes in invasive ventilation settings
- titration of non-invasive ventilation
- prior to major surgery as a baseline to facilitate post-operative comparison
- major trauma

Principles of ABG analysis

Oxygen supply to the tissues is dependent upon how oxygen disassociates itself from the haemoglobin (Hb) molecule to be made available for the tissues. This in turn is dependent upon blood pH, body temperature and $PaCO_2$ of the blood (Hubbard & Mechan 1997). As the blood becomes more acidotic, warmer and with a higher $PaCO_2$, the oxygen dissociation curve shifts to the right and reduces the Hb molecule's affinity for oxygen (Athern *et al.* 1995). Although less oxygen can be picked up by the lungs, more can be released to the tissues (Valenti *et al.* 1997). Conversely a shift to the left results in the Hb molecule having a greater affinity to oxygen but less can be released to the tissues. Therefore this may result in poor oxygenation despite an adequate PaO_2.

When a sample of arterial blood is processed by a blood gas analyser it provides not only an invaluable and accurate insight into the patient's respiratory function but also provides a window into their metabolic status.

The levels of blood gases are dependent upon three variables: blood supply, ventilation and diffusion. Therefore if there is a poor blood supply to the alveoli but adequate ventilation, insufficient diffusion will lead to a retention of PCO_2, e.g. pulmonary embolus. Conversely if there is a good blood supply to the alveoli but poor ventilation, gaseous exchange will also be compromised, e.g. COPD, pneumonia and asthma. Both of these imbalances will lead to a perfusion–ventilation (VQ) mismatch or a 'shunt' (Smyth 2005). Blood gas units of measurement are kilopascals (kPa) or millimetres of mercury (mmHg). Both units are currently in use (to convert kPa to mmHg: kPa $\times$ 7.5 = mmHg and to convert mmHg to kPa: mmHg $\div$ 7.5 = kPa).

Parameters measured by a blood gas analyser

- pH: 7.35–7.45. Measures overall acid–base balance of the blood sample (Pruitt & Jacobs 2004) and is affected by both respiratory and metabolic function (Woodrow 2004). Acid–base balance is the maintenance of hydrogen ion balance (H^+) that enables normal cell function (Simpson 2004). H^+ and pH levels have an inverse ratio, i.e. one increases as the other decreases (Simpson 2004). Small changes in pH are life threatening (Allen 2005) therefore the body relies on compensatory mechanisms to counteract dramatic changes in pH. Buffers in the body act as chemical sponges which absorb excess alkali or acid (Allen 2005).
- PaO_2: 10–13.3 kPa (75–100 mmHg). This is the measurement of partial pressure of oxygen dissolved in the blood sample, not how much oxygen is in the blood (UKRC 2004). Arterial PO_2 (PaO_2) is dependent on the alveolar PO_2 (PAO_2) (UKRC 2004).

Arterial PO_2 is always less than alveolar PO_2 and the extent of this difference is dependent upon the incidence of lung disease. Increases in the difference indicate VQ mismatch (Simpson 2004). A person with normal lungs breathing air (FiO_2 0.21) at sea level should have a PaO_2 of >11 kPa (80 mmHg) and breathing an oxygen concentration of 50% (FiO_2 0.5) at sea level will result in a PaO_2 of approximately 40 kPa (300 mmHg) (UKRC 2004). When a patient is receiving supplementary oxygen, a normal PaO_2 will not necessarily indicate adequate ventilation as small increases in FiO_2 will overcome any hypoxaemia caused by underventilation (UKRC 2004). A PaO_2 level of <8 kPa (60 mmHg) is considered a diagnosis of hypoxaemia (British Thoracic Society 2002). Critically ill patients have increased oxygen demands because of the pathological demands of the body (Shoulders-Odom 2000). It is critical that these increased oxygen demands are met to maintain adequate tissue oxygenation and prevent cell death.

- $PaCO_2$: 4.7–6.0 kPa (35–45 mmHg). This is the measurement of partial pressure of dissolved carbon dioxide in the blood (more soluble than oxygen). In order to be carried to the lungs to be exhaled carbon dioxide is transported in a plasma solution as carbonic acid (H_2CO_3). If the patient has too little or too much carbon dioxide this will have an effect on the acidity or alkalinity of the blood (Allen 2005). Carbon dioxide concentration provides information about the adequacy of ventilation (Allen 2005). Carbon dioxide is a waste product of tissue metabolism and the respiratory centres in the brainstem are stimulated in a response to high levels of carbon dioxide (Woodrow 2004). The respiratory centres in the brainstem are sensitive to hydrogen ion concentration (UKRC 2004). Therefore, as the carbon dioxide rises the respiratory centres are stimulated to increase respiratory rate and depth and reduce carbon dioxide levels, and conversely when there is hyperventilation and carbon dioxide reduces, the respiratory centres are stimulated to reduce respiratory rate and depth:

$$CO_2 + H_2O \quad = \quad H_2CO_3 \quad = \quad HCO_3^- + H^+$$

| carbon dioxide plus water | | carbonic acid | | bicarbonate plus hydrogen ions |

- Bicarbonate (HCO_3^-) (22–26 mmol/l). The major buffering systems in the body involve bicarbonate, protein and phosphate, however bicarbonate is the most important (Resuscitation Council UK 2006). Buffers have two qualities: they bind free hydrogen ions when they are in excess (acidosis) and donate hydrogen ions when they are too low (alkalosis) (Simpson 2004).

- Base excess (BE) (–2 mmol to +2 mmol). Base excess is the quantity of acid or base required to restore the blood to a pH of 7.4 (Resuscitation Council UK 2006; Woodrow 2004). A negative value indicates a deficit of base (or excess of acid) and a positive value indicates an excess of base (or deficit of acid) (Resuscitation Council UK 2006).

- SaO_2 (92–99%). Arterial oxygen saturation is the percentage of oxygen that has combined with the haemoglobin (Hb) molecule. Oxygen combines with Hb in sufficient amounts to meet the needs of the body, whilst at the same time releasing oxygen to meet tissue demands (Shoulders-Odom 2000).

- Other values: most analysers measure electrolytes, e.g. sodium (Na), potassium (K), calcium (Ca) and chloride (Cl), Hb and lactate, which can be useful for a 'quick check'. In most ICUs these values are accepted as accurate and treatment is titrated according to them. However, if aberrant values are obtained it will be necessary to obtain laboratory analysis for comparison.

Normal ranges for ABG analysis are shown in Table 3.3.

Table 3.3 Normal ranges for ABG results.

Parameter	Normal range
pH	7.35–7.45
PO_2	10.0–13.3 kPa
PCO_2	4.6–6.0 kPa
Bicarbonate (HCO_3^-)	22–26 mmol/l
SaO_2	>95%
Base excess	–2 to +2

© Sheila K. Adam and Sue Osborne 1997. Reproduced by permission of Oxford University Press from Adam & Osborne 1997.

Systematic analysis of ABG results

Driscoll *et al.* (1997) recommend three principles in analysing ABG results:

- Consider the patient's clinical history and physical examination.
- Systematically analyse the results.
- Integrate the clinical findings with interpretation of the data.

A systematic approach for the analysis of ABGs is a prerequisite for objective assessment and the UKRC suggest a five-step approach:

Step l: assess oxygenation

- Is the patient hypoxic?
- What supplementary oxygen are they receiving?

Step 2: determine pH level

Is there an acidosis (pH < 7.35) or alkalosis (pH > 7.45) present?

Step 3: determine the respiratory component

Is the $PaCO_2$ low (<4.7 kPa, <35 mmHg) or high (>6.0 kPa, >45 mmHg)? If the carbon dioxide is low this may indicate either a primary respiratory alkalosis or secondary respiratory compensation for a metabolic acidosis. If the carbon dioxide is high this may indicate either a primary respiratory acidosis or secondary compensation for a metabolic alkalosis.

Step 4: determine metabolic component

Is the bicarbonate low (<22 mmol/l) or high (>26 mmol/l)? If the bicarbonate is low this may indicate a primary metabolic acidosis or a secondary renal compensation for a respiratory alkalosis. If the bicarbonate is high this may indicate a primary metabolic alkalosis or a secondary metabolic compensation for a respiratory acidosis. It is not necessary to evaluate BE as the level of BE and bicarbonate mirror each other.

Step 5

Combine the findings from steps 2, 3 and 4 and determine what the primary disturbance is and whether there are any compensatory mechanisms evident.

Table 3.4 Summary of changes in acid–base disorders (Resuscitation Council UK 2006).

Acid–base disorder	pH	PaCO$_2$	HCO$_3^-$
Respiratory acidosis	↓	↑	N
Metabolic acidosis	↓	N	↓
Respiratory alkalosis	↑	↓	N
Metabolic alkalosis	↑	N	↑
Respiratory acidosis with metabolic compensation	↓*	↑	↑
Metabolic acidosis with respiratory compensation	↓*	↓	↓
Respiratory alkalosis with metabolic compensation	↑*	↓	↓
Metabolic alkalosis with respiratory compensation	↑*	↑	↑
Mixed metabolic and respiratory alkalosis	↓	↑	↓
Mixed metabolic and respiratory alkalosis	↑	↓	↑

*If the compensation is virtually complete the pH may be normal.

Best practice – arterial blood gas analysis

Consider the patient's clinical history and physical examination
Systematically analyse the results
Integrate the clinical findings with interpretation of the data
Never remove supplementary oxygen when taking an arterial blood sample for analysis. It is important to assess the patient's response to supplementary oxygen and the withholding of oxygen in the compromised patient is dangerous practice

---

The changes in acid–base disorders are summarised in Table 3.4.

Classification of imbalance

Acid–base balance disturbance occurs when there are either too many H$^+$ (acidosis) or too few (alkalosis) (Simpson 2004). If this imbalance has a respiratory cause the metabolic system will aim to compensate as will the respiratory system if there is a metabolic imbalance.

There are four classifications of imbalance with or without compensation:

- *respiratory* acidosis
- *metabolic* acidosis

- *respiratory* alkalosis
- *metabolic* alkalosis

Respiratory acidosis

Respiratory acidosis occurs when the pH of blood falls below 7.35 (Simpson 2004) and is caused by inadequate ventilation leading to the retention of carbon dioxide and an increase in free hydrogen ions. Predisposing factors include:

- exacerbation of COPD
- pulmonary oedema
- pneumonia
- mechanical disruption to ventilation, e.g. diaphragmatic rupture, fractured sternum
- neurological disorder, e.g. intracranial events and neuromuscular disorders
- over-sedation, i.e. opiates or sedatives
- self-poisoning

An example of respiratory acidosis without metabolic compensation:

pH 7.24
$PaCO_2$ 8.0 kPa (60 mmHg)
PaO_2 7.5 kPa (56 mmHg)
HCO_3^- 24 mmol/l
BE 0
SaO_2 94%

It is vital that there is a fine balance between acids and bases to provide the optimum neutral environment for cell function. In the above example, the buffer system provided by the kidneys should counterbalance the free H^+ ions as a result of excessive carbon dioxide production. Compensation for acidosis or alkalosis is achieved by the other system (i.e. the renal system will compensate for respiratory derangement and the respiratory system for metabolic derangement). The lungs however, provide a much quicker compensatory mechanism than the kidneys, which can take hours or even days to compensate adequately.

An example of respiratory acidosis with metabolic compensation:

pH 7.37
$PaCO_2$ 7.3 kPa (55 mmHg)
PaO_2 9.6 kPa (72 mmHg)
HCO_3^- 32 mmol/l
BE +6
SaO_2 95%

In this example there is an increase in the amount of HCO_3^- reabsorbed by the kidneys which act as a buffer for the excessive free H^+ ions. The compensation is only said to be adequate if the pH has returned to within normal limits, as in this example.

Metabolic acidosis

This involves excess fixed acid production, i.e. lactate or loss of HCO_3^-. Causes include:

- diarrhoea
- cardiac arrest
- diabetic ketoacidosis
- renal failure
- distributive shock
- salicylate poisoning

Example of metabolic acidosis without respiratory compensation:

pH 7.20
$PaCO_2$ 4.7 kPa (35 mmHg)
PaO_2 10.0 kPa (75 mmHg)
HCO_3^- 16 mmol/l
BE −12
SaO_2 96%

The lack of circulating HCO_3^- has resulted in a metabolic acidosis reflected in a base deficit of −12.

Example of metabolic acidosis with respiratory compensation:

pH 7.35
$PaCO_2$ 2.7 kPa (20 mmHg)
PaO_2 11.8 kPa (88 mmHg)
HCO_3^- 12 mmol/l

BE −14
SaO$_2$ 97%

The respiratory system has compensated by reducing the level of carbon dioxide by hyperventilation, thereby reducing the level of circulating free H$^+$ ions.

Respiratory alkalosis

Respiratory alkalosis is caused by the over-excretion of carbon dioxide leading to a reduction in free hydrogen ions and an alkalotic state. Predisposing factors include:

- hyperventilation in hysteria
- excessive mechanical ventilation

Example of respiratory alkalosis without metabolic compensation:

pH 7.50
PaCO$_2$ 2.5 kPa (19 mmHg)
PaO$_2$ 8.6 kPa (65 mmHg)
HCO$_3$$^-$ 22 mmol/l
BE +1
SaO$_2$ 92%

Example of respiratory alkalosis with metabolic compensation:

pH 7.44
PaCO$_2$ 2.6 kPa (19 mmHg)
PaO$_2$ 8.9 kPa (67 mmHg)
HCO$_3$$^-$ 15 mmol/l
BE −9
SaO$_2$ 93%

The patient excretes bicarbonate ions via the renal system in order to reduce the presence of alkaline buffers in the blood further.

Metabolic alkalosis

Metabolic alkalosis is caused by a loss of acids or an increase in alkaline buffers, i.e. bicarbonate. Causes include:

- gastrointestinal disorders, e.g. severe vomiting

- overdose of antacids
- diuretics

An example of metabolic alkalosis without respiratory compensation:

pH 7.67
$PaCO_2$ 4.2 kPa (31 mmHg)
PaO_2 13.1 kPa (97 mmHg)
HCO_3^- 38 mmol/l
BE +15
SaO_2 98%

There is an increase in circulating bicarbonate i.e. an excess of alkaline leading to an alkalosis.

An example of metabolic alkalosis with respiratory compensation:

pH 7.45
$PaCO_2$ 7.6 kPa (57 mmHg)
PaO_2 12.4 kPa (93 mmHg)
HCO_3^- 32 mmol/l
BE +4
SaO_2 96%

The respiratory system retains carbon dioxide in order to create more available free hydrogen ions to balance the excess alkaline production, thereby maintaining the equilibrium.

PRINCIPLES OF CAPNOGRAPHY

Measuring end-tidal carbon dioxide ($ETCO_2$) is helpful when monitoring the critically ill patient. There is virtually no carbon dioxide in inspired air; but as $ETCO_2$ concentration is very similar to arterial carbon dioxide partial pressure ($PaCO_2$), measuring $ETCO_2$ does provide an indication to the adequacy of ventilation (Leach 2004).

Capnometry is the measurement of expired carbon dioxide (Mosby 2006). It can simply be undertaken by attaching a colourimetric detector (Fig. 3.5) to the tracheal tube: a pH-sensitive indicator strip turns yellow in the presence of exhaled carbon dioxide, thus confirming correct tracheal tube placement

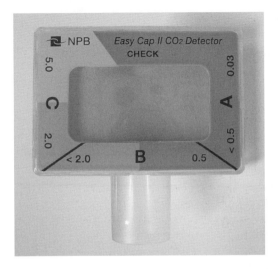

Fig. 3.5 A colourimetric carbon dioxide detector (Proact Medical Ltd).

(Andrews & Nolan 2006). This colourimetric detector device is frequently used during cardiopulmonary resuscitation to help ascertain that the tracheal tube has been inserted into the trachea. New capnography devices are now available for patients who are awake and spontaneously breathing (Fig. 3.6).

Electronic capnometry, using infrared light technology, is more accurate and reliable than colourimetric capnometry, particularly in patients with circulatory shock (Salem 2001). It works on the principle that carbon dioxide absorbs infrared light in proportion to its concentration (Gwinnutt 2006). It produces a capnogram, a waveform that shows the proportion of carbon dioxide in exhaled air (Mosby 2006). This method of monitoring is referred to as capnography.

The use of capnography has expanded over recent years and it is currently used in a variety of acute care settings. It provides comprehensive information on $ETCO_2$, with a continuous characteristic waveform (Fig. 3.7) being displayed (Andrews & Nolan 2006). It provides clinicians with information regarding ventilation and assists in clinical diagnosis, e.g. pulmonary embolism

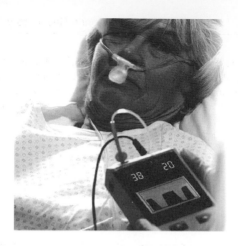

Fig. 3.6 A capnography device for use in a patient breathing spontaneously (Proact Medical Ltd).

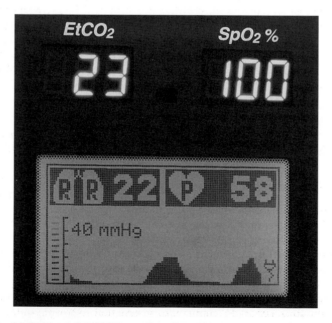

Fig. 3.7 A characteristic $EtCO_2$ waveform (Proact Medical Ltd).

(Ahrens & Sona 2003). It is particularly helpful in the critically ill patient because it can alert the nurse to hypoventilation even when the patient's pulse oximetry readings are normal (Woomer & Berkheimer 2003). Capnography is also a helpful monitoring tool if pulse oximetry is malfunctioning (Kober *et al.* 2004).

Indications for capnography include:

- respiratory monitoring in critically ill patients
- during the transport of critically ill patients
- during anaesthesia
- following tracheal tube insertion to confirm correct placement
  (Bersten 2004)

Changes in the waveform produced enable correlation with clinical conditions, e.g. airflow obstruction.

In patients with a low cardiac output or chest disease, the gap between the arterial carbon dioxide and $ETCO_2$ levels increases; care must therefore be taken when interpreting $ETCO_2$ concentrations in these circumstances (Gwinnutt 2006). Arterial blood gas analysis enables the $ETCO_2$ to be calibrated against the $PaCO_2$: the capnography can then be used as an indirect, continuous monitor of $PaCO_2$, and therefore ventilation (Andrews & Nolan 2006).

MONITORING PRIORITIES OF A VENTILATED PATIENT

Mechanical ventilation is a major supportive treatment for critically ill patients and as such is a frequent occurrence in the ICU (Newmarch 2006). The use of an endotracheal or tracheostomy tube ensures the delivery of guaranteed fraction of inspired oxygen (FiO_2) and delivery of gas under a pre-set constant pressure or at a pre-set tidal volume (Newmarch 2006).

There are many physical, as well as psychological, parameters to be monitored, all of which must be fully understood by the nurse caring for these patients. The primary physiological changes taking place concern the cardiovascular system. As mechanical ventilation (MV) is totally converse to normal physiological breathing, cardiovascular effects can be ongoing and therefore continuous, consistent monitoring is essential. During spontaneous breathing air is 'sucked in' under a negative pressure, whereas with MV air is delivered under a positive pressure (Manno 2005). As air is delivered under a positive pressure, venous return to the right side of the heart is impeded, reducing preload and, consequently, cardiac output (Manno 2005). In addition, the fall in cardiac output leads to a reduction in renal blood flow which stimulates the release of antidiuretic hormone (ADH) causing fluid retention and oedema.

The classification of ventilators depends upon the methods used to cycle from the inspiratory phase to the expiratory phase (Newmarch 2006). If the ventilator mode is pressure cycled, inspiratory pressure is set, rate is set and volume is dependent upon the patient's lung compliance. If the mode is volume cycled, the tidal volume is pre-set, rate is set and peak inspiratory pressure varies dependent upon the patient's degree of lung compliance. The most frequently used ventilator modes are listed below:

- *SIMV (volume or pressure cycled).* Synchronised intermittent mandatory ventilation delivers a pre-set volume or pressure, at a pre-set rate and is synchronised with the patient's own respiratory effort (Schumacher & Chernecky 2005). A comparison between the patient's breath and mandatory breaths will be demonstrated and should be recorded. This is the most commonly used ventilator mode and can be used as a weaning mode.
- *CMV controlled mandatory ventilation.* Delivers gas at a pre-set volume and rate and does not synchronise with spontaneous breaths (Manno 2005).
- *Pressure support ventilation (PSV).* Spontaneous mode where a pre-set inspiratory pressure augments the patient's breath. The patient controls the rate and volume of ventilation (Schumaker & Chernecky 2005).
- *Pressure control ventilation (PC).* Gas is delivered at a pre-set rate and inspiratory pressure and the volume is determined by the patient's lung compliance.
- *Bi-level positive airway pressure (BIPAP).* A pressure-controlled ventilation allows the patient to breathe spontaneously anywhere in the cycle and provides high and low positive end expiratory pressure (Manno 2005).

- *Continuous positive airway pressure (CPAP)*. Provides a constant positive airway pressure in spontaneous mode (frequently seen with PSV) and promotes gaseous exchange by opening alveoli and increasing functional residual capacity (Schumaker & Chernecky 2005).
- *Positive end expiratory pressure (PEEP)*. Same principle as CPAP but in non-spontaneous mode.

Parameters to be monitored during mechanical ventilation

During mechanical ventilation careful note should be taken of the following measurements, which should be recorded hourly and after any alterations in settings:

- *Respiratory rate*: the number of breaths delivered by the ventilator per minute (Manno 2005) and any spontaneous breaths.
- *Tidal volume (V_T)*: volume of air per expired breath. This should be the same or slightly more than the preset V_T. Aim for 6–8 ml/kg, i.e. maximum for a 70 kg person should be 560 ml per breath. A decrease in mortality has been demonstrated with patients with acute lung injury using these lower tidal volumes (Brower *et al.* 2000). If the inspired V_T does not correlate with the expired V_T in volume-cycled ventilation, check for leaks in the circuit, check that the cuff on the endotracheal tube is inflated sufficiently and check the ventilator (inner valves, etc.). If tidal volume (V_T) is high, the patient is probably breathing spontaneously. Increases in tidal volumes could also be due to added gas into the circuit, i.e. when nebulising drugs.
- *Minute volume (mv)*: amount exhaled each minute. It should always be the same as pre-set tidal volume multiplied by the pre-set rate ($V_T \times$ rate = mv).
- *Peak inspiratory pressure*: peak pressure at which the tidal volume is delivered or is pre-set in pressure-cycled ventilation. Measured in cmH_2O, it must always be at the lowest possible to ensure adequate ventilation. This will lessen the cardiovascular side effects of MV and reduce the risks of barotrauma.
- *PEEP*: positive end expiratory pressure. This should range between 5 and 20 cmH_2O. PEEP is over and above inspiratory pressure, i.e. if pressure is set at 20cmH_2O and PEEP at 5 cmH_2O, the peak inspiratory pressure will be 25 cmH_2O.

- *FiO$_2$*: fraction of inspired oxygen expressed as a fraction of a whole, i.e. 40% = FiO$_2$ 0.4.
- *Inspiratory to expiratory ratio (I:E ratio)*. Each breath has three components: inspiration, pause and expiration. Alteration of the I:E ratio manipulates alveolar gas exchange, normal I:E ratio is 1:2 (Newmarch 2006).
- *ETCO$_2$ levels* (if used).
- *Humidifier temperature*: should be 37°C at the patient end.
- Ensure all high and low alarm limits are set appropriately and monitored regularly.

> NEVER SILENCE A VENTILATOR ALARM UNLESS YOU ARE SURE OF THE CAUSE.

Monitoring the endotracheal tube
The following are key principles of the management of a patient with an endotracheal tube:

- Maintain patency: ventilation should be closely monitored and suction should be immediately available.
- Secure the endotracheal tube to the patient's face with either adhesive or cotton tape.
- Alter the position of the tube daily at the lips to prevent pressure ulceration.
- Document the length at which the tube is cut and tied at the lips and check regularly for migration from these markers.
- Ensure continuous ECG with respiratory waveform.
- Ensure continuous pulse oximetry to detect hypoxaemia.
- Apply regular endotracheal suction, either with or without hyperinflation, to prevent sputum retention and maintain patency of the tube.
- Regularly auscultate for breath sounds to ensure equal inflation. The possibility of the tip of the tracheal tube slipping into the right main bronchus causing unilateral ventilation can therefore be excluded.
- Regular oral toilet, preferably with a soft toothbrush and toothpaste, will help to maintain oral hygiene and prevent proliferation of bacteria.

- Secure/support ventilator tubing to prevent excess weight on the endotracheal tube.
- Check emergency equipment, i.e. intubation equipment, suction and manual re-breathe circuits at least once a shift in case of accidental extubation.
- Use endotracheal tubes with high-volume, low-pressure cuffs to minimise the risk of tracheal stenosis/ischaemia and regularly check cuff pressures with cuff manometers.

The nurse should be alert to the possible complications of endotracheal intubation. The acronym DOPE is helpful in detecting problems:

Displacement of tube
Obstruction of tube
Pneumothorax
Equipment

Other complications of tracheal intubation include oesophageal or right main bronchus intubation, herniation of the cuff, damage to vocal cords, tracheal stenosis, tracheal ulceration and damage to soft palate and lips.

MONITORING THE PATIENT RECEIVING NON-INVASIVE VENTILATION (NIV)

The use of NIV to avoid endotracheal intubation was first described in 1989 (Keenan *et al.* 2005). It has now become a frequent occurrence in ICUs, HDUs and wards primarily to avoid the use of invasive ventilation. There are many different terminologies which describe NIV depending on machines used (Woodrow 2003): continuous positive airway pressure (CPAP), non-invasive positive pressure ventilation (NIPPV), nasal ventilation (NV), and the most frequently used bi-level positive airway pressure (BiPAP®). The British Thoracic Society recommends the term NIV, which incorporates all of the above (BTS 2002).

NIV is delivered via a face or nasal mask and is predominantly used for the exacerbation of COPD (Woodrow 2003). NIV gives the patient breathing assistance by delivering a pressured gas through a tight-fitting mask (Preston 2001). By supporting patients with NIV, work of breathing is reduced, tidal volume is increased and oxygenation and hypercapnia improves (Preston 2001). Bi-level NIV consists of the following parameters:

- Inspiratory positive airway pressure (IPAP)
- Expiratory positive airway pressure (EPAP)

BTS guidelines (2002) recommend the use of bi-level NIV for:

- COPD with respiratory acidosis (pH 7.25–7.35)
- hypercapnic respiratory failure secondary to chest wall deformity, e.g. scoliosis, thoracoplasty, neuromuscular disease
- cardiogenic pulmonary oedema that is unresponsive to CPAP alone
- weaning patients from mechanical ventilation

Bi-level NIV alternates between inspired positive airway pressure (IPAP) and expired positive airway pressure (EPAP). The higher level of inspiratory pressure occurs during inspiration (IPAP) and increases tidal volume, helping to reduce carbon dioxide levels and reduce the work of breathing (Woodrow 2003). The lower level of pressure occurs at the end of expiration (EPAP) maintaining a positive pressure, thereby recruiting alveoli and preventing atelectasis to improve oxygenation (Woodrow 2003). Typical pressures to commence bi-level NIV would be IPAP of $12\,cmH_2O$ and EPAP of $5\,cmH_2O$, titrated according to the patient's response.

When monitoring a patient receiving bi-level NIV the following precautions should be observed:

- Take ABGs after 1 hour, some improvement should be recognised. If carbon dioxide levels and respiratory acidosis have not significantly improved in 4–6 hours invasive ventilation should be commenced (BTS 2002).
- Monitor vital signs regularly, continuous SpO_2 is vital (Preston 2001).
- Monitor and record levels of IPAP, EPAP, respiratory rate, FiO_2, tidal volume and minute volume.
- Administer regular eye and mouth care as high-pressure gas can be very drying.
- Be aware that the masks can be claustrophobic for some patients. When condition has stabilised, regular breaks from

the mask for oral toilet, diet and fluids can be given, but supplementary oxygen must be administered.

- Monitor chest wall movement (BTS 2002).

PRINCIPLES OF MONITORING A PATIENT WITH A CHEST DRAIN

A chest drain can be used to manage a variety of thoracic
conditions. It can safely remove air (pneumothorax) or fluid
(haemothorax, pleural effusion) from the pleural cavity and
prevent its reintroduction, allowing the lungs to re-expand
(Hilton 2004).

The drain insertion site is determined by whether air or fluid
requires removal. Air usually rises to the apex of the lung and is
therefore most efficiently removed when the tip of the drain is
anterior and apical to the chest cavity (Avery 2000). The safest
insertion site is in the mid-axillary line, second intercostal space
(BTS 2002). On the other hand fluid usually collects at the base of
the lung and is therefore most efficiently removed when the drain
is posterior and basal to the chest cavity at the fourth, fifth or
sixth intercostal space.

When monitoring a patient with a chest drain the following
precautions should be observed:

- Monitor the patient's vital signs, in particular in relation to the
  patient's respiratory status.
- Request a chest radiograph following insertion of chest drain
  to check its position and ensure the lung has re-inflated (BTS
  2002).
- Administer prescribed analgesia for pain (Hilton 2004).
- Secure the drain to prevent movement, however large
  amounts of tape and dressing are unnecessary and a transparent dressing and one anchor tape are recommended (BTS
  2002).
- Regularly check the fluid level, as an underwater sealed drain
  operates as a one-way valve allowing air to bubble out through
  the water during expiration and coughing but not permitting
  air to be drawn back in (Avery 2000).
- Observe and record the amount, consistency and colour of any
  drainage. If drainage is collecting in a fluid-dependent loop of

the tubing either reposition or shorten the tube to prevent it from occurring (preferable) or regularly lift and drain the tubing (Schmelz *et al.* 1999).

- Observe the level of water in the tubing. It should fluctuate with respirations; a gradual decrease in fluctuation could indicate re-expansion of the lung while a sudden decrease suggests that the tube is blocked (Avery 2000). Bubbling is another sign that air is being evacuated from the pleural space; it should decrease as the lung reinflates. The continuation of bubbling suggests a continued leak in the visceral pleura (BTS 2002). Also check that there are no loose connections in the system. If a blocked tube is suspected, check that the cause is not a kinked tube. The tubing may need to be replaced. 'Milking' the tube is not recommended as this causes unnecessary fluctuations in intrapleural pressures.

- Monitor any suction used; low-grade suction can be used to help remove air or fluid from the chest cavity. However insufficient suction will prevent lung expansion, increasing the risk of tension pneumothorax (Avery 2000) while too much suction can lead to air and oxygen being 'sucked out' leading to hypoxia (Tang *et al.* 1999). A suction pressure of 10–20 cmH$_2$O is normally used (McManus 1998). N.B. If a chest drain is connected to a suction unit which has been switched off it is equivalent to it being clamped off and could therefore result in a tension pneumothorax (Mallett & Dougherty 2000).

- Clamp the drain close to the chest wall only when changing the bottle/container or after accidental disconnection. A bubbling chest drain should never be clamped (BTS 2002).

- Ensure the drainage bottle is kept below the level of the patient's chest to prevent fluid re-entering the pleural space (Avery 2000).

- Monitor the chest drain insertion site for signs of infection.

PRINCIPLES OF MONITORING THE PATIENT WITH A TEMPORARY TRACHEOSTOMY

A tracheostomy is an opening in the anterior wall of the trachea below the cricoid cartilage (Russell 2005). Patients who require a temporary tracheostomy are a frequent occurrence in the critically ill population both within critical care units and during their recovery phase in ward areas. Insertion of a tracheostomy tube is a surgical procedure which is performed either in the operating theatre (surgical tracheostomy) or in the ICU (percutaneous dilational tracheostomy).

Indications for a temporary tracheostomy include:

- mechanical upper airway obstruction (Russell & Matta 2004)
- trauma to tongue or mandible (Seay *et al.* 2002)
- elective head and neck surgery (Russell & Matta 2004)
- prolonged oral intubation (>14 days)
- inability to wean from mechanical ventilation
- inability to maintain own airway
- severe burns of head and neck (Seay *et al.* 2002)

Monitoring priorities of the patient with a temporary tracheostomy

A patient who has been in intensive care and subsequently required a temporary tracheostomy will often have suffered a severe and protracted illness resulting in severe debilitation. These patients will have significantly impaired muscle strength and physical energy reserve and remain susceptible to infection. Therefore, these vulnerable patients require continuous monitoring in the post intensive care period. Monitoring should focus on maintaining the patency of the tracheostomy tube and the early detection of complications which may occur. A tracheostomy tube which has a removable inner tube for cleaning purposes can significantly reduce the serious complication of a blocked tube and compromised airway (Russell 2005).

Monitoring principles are listed below:

- Continual observation: ensure the patient is located in a highly visible area of the ward.
- Monitor the position and patency of the tube: continually observe the patient for signs of respiratory distress, ensuring they have access to call buttons and communication aids.
- Regular physiological monitoring: respiratory rate, heart rate, blood pressure, SpO_2, temperature.

- Monitor the temperature and water level of the humidifier, ensuring water traps are empty and positioned lower than the head height of the patient.
- Observe and record the amount, colour and consistency of secretions on tracheal suction (2–4-hourly dependent upon individual requirements) (Edgtton-Winn & Wright 2005).
- Observe the amount and consistency of sputum in the inner tube when cleaned and clean according to requirements (at *least* three times per day).
- Monitor microbiological results from sputum samples.
- Monitor nutritional status; keep a food diary if not receiving enteral nutrition.
- Regularly observe the tracheal stoma for signs of infection, such as redness or malodorous discharge.

Best practice – temporary tracheostomies

Have available at the bedside a tracheostomy tube of the same size and type which the patient has in situ and a size below (Seay *et al.* 2002)

Have available at the bedside tracheal dilating forceps

Ensure the tracheostomy tube is securely fixed with tape and regularly changed, particularly if soiled

Clean the tracheostomy site with saline as required and always with two nurses

Use sterile technique for suctioning the tracheostomy tube and wear protective clothing (Russell 2005)

Be aware of emergency procedures if the tube becomes dislodged including appropriate details of personnel to contact

Be aware of who has overall responsibility for the management of the tracheostomy (e.g. ear, nose and throat (ENT) team)

Ensure that the tracheostomy tube is changed according to hospital policy by trained practitioners

Utilise a tracheostomy chart (Fig. 3.8) which monitors the patient's progress towards decannulation

Ensure emergency equipment is at the bedside, i.e. a re-breathe circuit with both a catheter mount and a face mask for emergencies (Edgtton-Winn & Wright 2005)

Name...Unit number.............................

Date of tracheostomy......................................Tube size/type..........................

Criteria for use of purple cap (all must be Yes)

Relevant multidisciplinary team members aware	Yes/No
Oxygen saturations maintained ie 92--95%	Yes/No
Strong spontaneous cough	Yes/No
Cuff is deflated	Yes/No
Patient aware of procedure	Yes/No
Fenestrated tube with inner tube	Yes/No
Tube has been downsized	Yes/No

Weaning process

Day 1	Discuss -- Apply cap at 08:00 for up to 12 hours, give humidified oxygen by mouth if required. Remove cap overnight. Monitor respiratory rate and saturations 10 minutes after occlusion and hourly for first 4 hours -- then 4 hourly. Re-apply cap following suction via tracheostomy.
Day 2	Cap from 08:00 as above plan to occlude during daylight hours if tolerated. Discuss with physiotherapists or OR team. Monitor respiratory rate and saturations 4 hourly.
Day 3	If cap is tolerated for daylight hours discuss with multidisciplinary team ie. medical team, physiotherapists and OR team re: decannulation. <u>Tracheostomy to be removed by a practitioner who has achieved the tracheostomy competencies</u>, a dry dressing and non-porous tape, i.e. sleek, applied over the stoma until healed. Inform Speech Therapist re: swallowing assessment.

Date/ Time	Speaking valve ON	Speaking valve OFF	Cap ON	Cap OFF	Comments	Signed

<u>REMOVE CAP IMMEDIATELY IF:</u>

- Patient becomes breathless and/or distressed
- Patient becomes sweaty or clammy
- Saturations drop to a level lower than before capping
- Patient requires frequent suction to clear secretions
- Patient becomes confused and/or agitated

Fig. 3.8 Tracheostomy weaning chart.

SCENARIOS

Scenario 1: type 1 respiratory failure

Damien, a 22-year-old man, was involved in a motorcycle accident in which he was in collision with a car. On clinical and radiological examination in the Emergency Department he was found to have fractured ribs, 5th, 6th, 7th and 8th on the right side and 4th and 5th on the left, causing a flail segment with paradoxical chest movements. A computed tomography (CT) scan of head and spine eliminated cervical spine or head injury.

Observations were: blood pressure (BP) 90/60, pulse 100, respirations 36/min, core temperature 35.8°C. He was commenced on high-flow oxygen at 15 l/min via a non re-breathe bag and aggressive fluid resuscitation was commenced. Continuous ECG monitoring, pulse oximetry were initiated and BP recordings were taken every 15 minutes. Blood was taken for a full biochemical, haematological screen, group and save and arterial blood gas analysis:

pH 7.37
$PaCO_2$ 4.0 kPa (30 mmHg)
PaO_2 5.5 kPa (41 mmHg)
HCO_3^- 24 mmol/l
BE −1
SaO_2 85%

What do these results demonstrate?
Blood gas analysis demonstrates a type 1 respiratory failure, resulting in severe hypoxaemia in the absence of carbon dioxide retention.

Despite the insertion of a thoracic nerve block for pain control, Damien continued to progress into severe type 1 respiratory failure and was electively intubated and ventilated in the Emergency Department. He was then transferred to ICU. Sedation and analgesia were provided with intravenous midazolam and morphine. On arrival to the ICU, MV was commenced at the following settings:

Mode: CMV (controlled mandatory ventilation)
VT: 455 ml (calculated at 6–8 ml/kg)
Rate: 12 breaths per minute
FiO_2: ·7
PEEP: + 7

Arterial blood gas analysis was repeated after 30 minutes at these ventilator settings:

pH 7.44
$PaCO_2$ 3.8 kPa (28.5 mmHg)
PaO_2 11.5 kPa (86 mmHg)
HCO_3^- 24
BE −2
SaO_2 96%

Damien's oxygenation has significantly improved with mechanical ventilation although he is still requiring significant concentrations of oxygen.

Sedation was titrated to a level which ensured that Damien could tolerate the ventilator but also so he could be roused by voice and was able to communicate using non-verbal methods. This enabled staff to measure the efficacy of his pain control using a visual analogue pain rating scale and allay his anxieties through orientating him to his environment and circumstances.

He continued to make progress over the following days and on day 7 Damien was successfully weaned from the ventilator and extubated. Effective pain control was achieved with the use of oral opioids and spontaneous respiration (with supplementary humidified oxygen) did not present any difficulties to him. He was discharged from ICU the following day and made an uneventful recovery thereafter.

Scenario 2: type 2 respiratory failure

Richard, a 67-year-old man with a known history of emphysema, presented with increasing breathlessness after a 'flu like' illness. On admission to the Emergency Department he was acutely breathless, centrally cyanosed and drowsy. Blood gas analysis was:

pH 7.11
$PaCO_2$ 10.8 kPa (81 mmHg)
PaO_2 6.8 kPa (51 mmHg)
HCO_3^- 32
BE +5
SaO_2 84%

What do these results tell you?
Blood gas analysis demonstrates a severe type 2 respiratory failure resulting in hypoxaemia, carbon dioxide retention and severe respiratory acidosis without metabolic compensation.

Continued

A chest radiograph (CXR) demonstrated a typical COPD appearance and a right middle lobe collapse. Richard was commenced on humidified oxygen at 40%, venous access was established and isotonic fluids prescribed at 100 ml/hr. Due to the history of rapid deterioration, purulent sputum, fever and left-sided chest pain, pneumonia was suspected and Richard was commenced on amoxicillin 1 g every 6 hours, azithromycin 500 mg IV daily and regular nebulised salbutamol, pulmicort and ipratroprium. As Richard was severely dyspnoeic he agreed to the insertion of a urinary catheter. At this time Richard was considered suitable for admission to a respiratory medical ward for ongoing conservative management. He was reviewed 1 hour later and arterial blood gases taken:

pH 7.10
$PaCO_2$ 11.1 kPa (83 mmHg)
PaO_2 7.3 kPa (55 mmHg)
HCO_3^- 33
BE +5
SaO_2 85%

What do these results tell you?
Blood gas analysis demonstrates an improvement in the PaO_2 but a further rise in $PaCO_2$ worsening the respiratory acidosis.

The increase in $PaCO_2$ indicates that the patient's condition might be deteriorating. In view of his past chronic medical history, his dependence upon home oxygen and the progressive nature of emphysema, it was decided that Richard was not a suitable candidate for invasive ventilation. He was therefore commenced on non-invasive ventilation: BiPAP (bi-level positive airway pressure ventilation) via a nasal mask. During BiPAP the patient continues to breathe spontaneously but is assisted by the ventilator. An upper pressure level is set (IPAP) and a lower pressure level set (EPAP). The ventilator then supports the patient's breath to these two set levels. This results in a reduction in the work of breathing, an increase in tidal volumes, an improvement in oxygenation and a reduction in $PaCO_2$. This non-invasive method is a simpler, cost-effective alternative, avoiding the significant risks associated with invasive ventilation, e.g. cardiovascular instability. Within an hour Richard's clinical condition was showing some improvement:

pH 7.19
$PaCO_2$ 9.0 kPa (67.5 mmHg)

PaO_2 8.1 kPa (61 mmHg)
HCO_3^- 34
BE +4
SaO_2 89%

What do these results tell you?

Blood gas analysis demonstrates an improvement in PaO_2 and a significant reduction in $PaCO_2$. The respiratory acidosis persists but is slowly resolving.

Richard continued to receive BiPAP for the next 3 days and with the aid of antibiotics, diuretics and physiotherapy was able to return home without the need for an ICU admission and invasive ventilation.

Scenario 3: type 2 respiratory failure

Chris, a 22-year-old man suffering from Duchenne muscular dystrophy, was admitted to an acute medical ward with a chest infection. On admission he was anxious, but co-operative. Oxygen 40% was being administered via a venturi mask. BP was 120/80, heart rate 100, respiratory rate 26/min and SpO_2 of 96%. He was being treated with broad-spectrum antibiotics and a dextrose saline infusion had been commenced at 100 ml/hr. Six hours later he became progressively more drowsy and difficult to rouse. His respiratory effort remained unchanged and his SpO_2 was 97%. He looked flushed but was apyrexial. Arterial blood gas results were as follows:

pH 7.21
$PaCO_2$ 10.6 kPa (79.5 mmHg)
PaO_2 9.6 kPa (72 mmHg)
HCO_3^- 22
BE +1
SaO_2 97%

What do these results tell you?

Blood gas analysis demonstrates a severe respiratory acidosis without metabolic compensation. This example demonstrates one limitation of pulse oximetry: a normal SpO_2 does not necessarily correlate with adequate ventilation.

CONCLUSION

Monitoring respiratory function requires accurate assessment of the efficacy of breathing, work of breathing and adequacy of ventilation together with a comprehensive patient assessment. Peak expiratory flow rate measurements, pulse oximetry and arterial blood gas analysis also contribute to the monitoring process.

REFERENCES

Adam, S. & Osborne, S. (1997) *Critical Care Nursing: Science and Practice*. Oxford University Press, Oxford.

Ahrens, T. & Sona, C. (2003) Capnography application in acute and critical care. *AACN Clinical Issues* **14** (2), 123–132.

Allen, K. (2005) Four step method of interpreting arterial blood gas analysis. *Nursing Times* **101** (1), 42.

Andrews, F. & Nolan, J. (2006) Critical care in the emergency department: monitoring the critically ill patient. *Emergency Medicine Journal* **23**, 561–564.

Athern, J., Fildes, S. & Peters, R. (1995) A guide to blood gases. *Nursing Standard* **9** (49), 50–52.

Avery, S. (2000) Insertion and management of chest drains. *Nursing Times Plus* **96** (37), 3–6.

Bennett, C. (2003) Nursing the breathless patient. *Nursing Standard* **17** (17), 45–53.

Berge, K.H., Lanier, W.L. & Scanlon, P.D. (1988) Ischaemic digital skin necrosis: a complication of the reusable nelcor pulse oximeter probe. *Anesthesia and Analgesia* **67**, 712–713.

Bersten, A. (2004) Respiratory monitoring. In: Bersten, A. & Soni, N., eds *Oh's Intensive Care Manual* 5th edn. Butterworth Heinemann, Oxford.

Blackwell, B. (1998) The practice and perception of intensive care staff using the closed suctioning system. *Journal of Advances in Nursing* **28** (5), 1020–1029.

Booker, R. (2004) The effective assessment of acute breathlessness in a patient. *Nursing Times* **100** (24), 61.

Brandt, M. *et al.* (1994) The paediatric chest tube. *Clinical Intensive Care* **5** (3), 123–129.

Brewis, R.A. (1996) *Respiratory Medicine*. W.B. Saunders, Philadelphia.

British Thoracic Society (2002) Non-invasive ventilation in acute respiratory failure. *Thorax* **57** (3), 192–211.

Brock-Utne, J.G., Botz, G. & Jaffe, R.A. (1992) Perioperative corneal abrasions. *Anaesthesiology* **77**, 221.

Brower, R., Matthay, M., Morris, A. *et al.* (2000) Ventilation with lower tidal volumes as compared with traditional tidal volumes for acute lung injury and the acute respiratory distress syndrome. *New England Journal of Medicine* **342** (18), 1301–1308.

Brower, R., Shanholtz, C., Fessler, H. *et al.* (1999) Prospective RCT comparing traditional vs reduced VT ventilation in acute respiratory distress syndrome patients. *Critical Care Medicine* **27** (8), 1492–1498.

Buist, M.D., Jarmolowski, E., Burton, P. *et al.* (1999) Recognising clinical instability in hospital patients before cardiac arrest or unplanned admission to intensive care. *Medical Journal of Australia* **324**, 22–25.

Carroll, P. (1991) What's new in chest tube management. *Registered Nurse* **54** (5), 35–40.

Carroll, P. (1998) Preventing noscomial pneumonia. *Registered Nurse* **61** (6), 44–48.

Coleman, M.D. & Coleman, N.A. (1996) Drug induced methaemoglobinaemia: treatment issues. *Drug Safety* **14** (6), 394–405.

Comroe, J.H. & Botelho, S. (1947) The unreliability of cyanosis in the recognition of arterial anoxaemia. *American Journal of Medical Science* **214**, 1–5.

Considine, J. (2005) The role of nurses in preventing adverse events related to respiratory dysfunction: literature review. *Journal of Advanced Nursing* **49** (6), 624–633.

Cote, C.J., Goldstein, A., Fuchsman, W.H. *et al.* (1988) The effect of nail polish on pulse oximetry. *Anesthesia and Analgesia* **67**, 683–686.

Crispin, C. & Daffurn, K. (2000) Nurses' response to acute severe illness. *Australian Critical Care* **11**, 131–133.

Davidson, J.A. & Hosie, H.E. (1993) Limitations of pulse oximetry: respiratory insufficiency – a failure of detection. *British Medical Journal* **307** (6900), 372–373.

Dobson, F. (1993) Shedding light on pulse oximetry. *Nursing Standard* **7** (46), 4–11.

Driscoll, P., Brown, T., Gwinnutt, C. *et al.* (1997) *A Simple Guide to Blood Gas Analysis.* BMJ Publishing Group, London.

Edgtton-Winn, M. & Wright, K. (2005) Tracheostomy: a guide to nursing care. *Australian Nursing Journal* **13** (5), 17–20.

Fieselman, J.F., Hendryx, M.S., Helms, C.M. *et al.* (1993) Respiratory rate predicts cardiopulmonary arrest for internal medicine patients. *Journal of General Internal Medicine* **8**, 354–360.

Fox, N. (2002) Pulse oximetry. *Nursing Times* **98** (40), 65–67.

Giuliano, K.K. (2006) Knowledge of pulse oximetry among critical care nurses. *Dimensions of Critical Care Nursing* **25** (1), 44–49.

Giuliano, K.K. & Higgins, T.L. (2005) New generation pulse oximetry in the care of critically ill patients. *American Journal of Critical Care* **14** (1), 26–37.

Godden, J. & Hiley, C. (1998) Managing the patient with a chest drain: a review. *Nursing Standard* **12** (32), 35–39.

Goldhill, D.R., White, S.A. & Sumner, A. (1999) Physiological values and procedures in the 24 hours before ICU admission from the ward. *Anaesthesia* **54**, 529–534.

Graham, A. (1996) Chest drain insertion. 'How to' Guide Series. *Care of the Critically Ill* **12** (5).

Gwinnutt, C. (2006) *Clinical Anaesthesia* 2nd edn. Blackwell Publishing, Oxford.

Hanning, C.D. & Alexander-Williams, J.M. (1995) Pulse oximetry: a practical review. *British Medical Journal* **311**, 367–370.

Harrahill, M. (1991) Pulse oximetry, pearls and pitfalls. *Journal of Emergency Nursing* **17** (6), 437–439.

Higgins, D. (2005) Pulse oximetry. *Nursing Times* **101** (6), 34.

Hilton, P. (2004) Evaluating the treatment options for spontaneous pneumothorax. *Nursing Times* **100** (28), 32.

Hinds, C.J. & Watson, D. (1996) *Intensive Care, a concise textbook* 2nd edn. W.B. Saunders, London.

Hubbard, J. & Mechan, D. (1997) *The Physiology of Health and Illness with Related Anatomy.* Stanley Thorn, Cheltenham.

Hutton, P. & Clutton-Brock, T. (1993) The benefits and pitfalls of pulse oximetry. *British Medical Journal* **307**, 457–458.

Jenson, L.A., Onyskiw, J.E. & Prasad, N.G.N. (1998) Meta-analysis of arterial oxygenation saturation monitoring by pulse oximetry in adults. *Heart and Lung* **27** (6), 387–408.

Jevon, P. & Ewens, B. (2000) Pulse oximetry. *Nursing Times* **96** (26), 43–44.

Jevon, P., Ewens, B. & Manzie, J. (2000) Peak flow. *Nursing Times* **96** (38), 49–50.

Jevon, P. & Ewens, B. (2001) Assessment of a breathless patient. *Nursing Standard* **15** (16), 48–53.

Johnson, N. (1987) *Respiratory Medicine.* Blackwell Scientific Publications, Oxford.

Keenan, S., Kernerman, P.D. & Cook, D.J.C. (1997) The effect of positive pressure ventilation on mortality in patients admitted with acute respiratory failure: a metaanalysis. *Critical Care Medicine* **25** (10), 1685–1692.

Keenan, S.P., Powers, C.E. & McCormack, D.G. (2005) Noninvasive positive-pressure ventilation in patients with milder chronic obstructive pulmonary disease exacerbations: a randomised controlled trial. *Respiratory Care* **50** (5), 610–616.

Kober, A., Schubert, B., Bertalanffy, P. *et al.* (2004) Capnography in non-tracheally intubated emergency patients as an additional tool in pulse oximetry for prehospital monitoring of respiration. *Anesthesia & Analgesia* **98** (1), 206–210.

Law, C. (2000) A guide to assessing sputum. *Nursing Times* **96** (24), Respiratory Care Supplement 7–10.

Leach, R. (2004) *Critical Care Medicine at a Glance.* Blackwell Publishing, Oxford.

Lowton, K. (1999) Pulse oximeters for the detection of hypoxaemia. *Professional Nurse* **14** (5), 343–350.

Lynne, M., Scnapp, M.D., Neal, H. *et al*. (1990) Pulse oximetry: uses and abuses. *Chest* **98**, 1244–1250.

Mackreth, B. (1990) Assessing pulse oximetry in the field. *Journal of Emergency Medical Services* **15**, 56–57, 59–60.

Mallett, J. & Dougherty, L. (2000) eds. *The Royal Marsden Hospital Manual of Clinical Nursing Procedures*. Blackwell Science, Oxford.

Manno, M.S. (2005) Managing mechanical ventilation. *Nursing* **35** (12), 36–41.

Mathews, P.J. (2005) The latest in respiratory care. *Nursing Management, Supplement: Critical Care Choices* **18**, 20–21.

McEnroe Ayers, D.M. & Stucky Lappin, J. (2004) Act fast when your patient has dyspnoea. *Nursing* **34** (7), 36–41.

McGloin, H., Adam, S.K. *et al*. (1999) Unexpected deaths and referrals to intensive care of patients on general wards. Are some cases potentially preventable? *Journal of the Royal College of Physicians* **33** (3), 255–259.

McManus, K. (1998) Chest drainage systems. 'How to' Guide Series. *Care of the Critically Ill* **14** (4).

Middleton, S. & Middleton, P.G. (1998) Assessment. In: Pryor, J.A. & Webber, B.A., eds *Physiotherapy for Respiratory and Cardiac Problems*. Churchill Livingstone, Edinburgh.

Miller, A. & Harvey, J. (1993) Guidelines for the management of spontaneous pneumothorax. Standards of Care Committee, British Thoracic Society. *British Medical Journal* **307** (6896), 114–117.

Miller, M. (2005) Changes in measuring peak expiratory flow. *Practice Nursing* **16** (10), 449–503.

Mosby (2006) *Mosby's Medical Dictionary* 7th edn. Mosby, USA.

Newmarch, C. (2006) Caring for the mechanically ventilated patient: part 2. *Nursing Standard* **20** (18), 55–64.

Nunn, A.J. & Gregg, I. (1989) New regression equations for predicting peak expiratory flow in adults. *British Medical Journal* **298**, 1068–1070.

Partridge, M. (1997) *Asthma Care; a Guide to Peak Flow*. Allen & Hanburys, Uxbridge.

Pierce, L. (1995) *Guide to Mechanical Ventilation and Intensive Respiratory Care*. W.B. Saunders, London.

Place, B. (1998) Pulse oximetry in adults. *Nursing Times* **94** (50), 48–49.

Place, B. (2000) Pulse oximetry: benefits and limitations. *Nursing Times* **96** (26), 42.

Preston, R. (2001) Introducing non-invasive positive pressure ventilation. *Nursing Standard* **15** (26), 42–45.

Pruitt, W.C. & Jacobs, M. (2004) Interpreting arterial blood gases: easy as ABC. *Nursing Times* **34** (8), 50–53.

Ralston, A.C. *et al*. (1991) Potential errors in pulse oximetry. *Anaesthesia* **46** (4), 291–295.

Rees, J. & Price, J.F. (1999) *ABC of Asthma*. BMJ Books, London.

Resuscitation Council UK (2006) *Advanced Life Support* 5th edn. Resuscitation Council UK, London.

Reynolds, K.J. *et al.* (1993) The effect of dyshemoglobins on pulse oximetry: Part 1, Theoretical approach & Part 2, Experimental results using an *in vitro* test system. *Journal of Clinical Monitoring* **9** (2), 81–90.

Rich, K. (1999) Inhospital cardiac arrest: pre-event variables and nursing response. *Clinical Nurse Specialist* **13** (3), 147–155.

Richardson, N.G.B. & Hale, J.E. (1995) Pulse oximetry – an unusual complication. *British Journal of Intensive Care* **5** (10), 326–327.

Ross-Plummer, B. (2000) Preparing patients with asthma for discharge. *Nursing Times* **96**, 24 Ntplus 13–15.

Russell, C. (2005) Providing the nurse with a guide to tracheostomy care and management. *British Journal of Nursing* **14** (8), 428–433.

Russell, C. & Matta, B. (2004) *Tracheostomy. A multi professional handbook.* Greenwich Medical Ltd, London UK.

Salem, M. (2001) Verification of endotracheal tube position. *Anesthesiology Clinics of North America* **19**, 813–839.

Schein, R.M.H., Hazday, N., Pena, M. *et al.* (1990) Clinical antecedents to in-hospital cardiac arrest. *Chest* **98**, 1388–1392.

Schmelz, J. *et al.* (1999) Effects of position of chest drainage tube on volume drained and pressure. *American Journal of Critical Care* **8** (5), 319–323.

Schnapp, L.M. & Cohen, N.H. (1990) Pulse oximetry: uses and abuses. *Chest* **98**, 1244–1250.

Schumacher, L. & Chernecky, C.C. (2005) *Real World Nursing Survival Guide: Critical Care and Emergency Nursing.* Saunders.

Seay, S.J., Gay, S.L. & Strauss, M. (2002) Tracheostomy emergencies. *Australian Journal of Nursing* **102** (3), 59–63.

Severinghaus, J.W. & Koh, S.O. (1990) Effect of anaemia on pulse oximetry accuracy at low saturation. *Journal of Clinical Monitoring* **6**, 85–88.

Shoulders-Odom, B. (2000) Using an algorithm to interpret arterial blood gases. *Dimensions of Critical Care Nursing* **19** (1), 36.

Simpson, H. (2004) Interpretation of arterial blood gases: a clinical guide for nurses. *British Journal of Nursing* **13** (9), 522–528.

Simpson, H. (2006) Respiratory assessment. *British Journal of Nursing* **15** (9), 484–488.

Smith, R. & Olson, M. (1989) Drug induced methaemoglobinaemia on pulse oximetry and mixed venous oximetry. *Anaesthesiology* **70**, 112–117.

Smyth, M. (2005) Acute respiratory failure: Part 2. Failure of ventilation: Exploring the other cause of acute respiratory failure. *American Journal of Nursing* **105** (6), 72AA–72DD.

Stoneham, M.D. *et al.* (1994) Knowledge about pulse oximetry amongst medical and nursing staff. *The Lancet* **344**, 1339–1342.

Tang, A. *et al.* (1999) A regional survey of chest drains: evidence-based practice? *Postgraduate Medical Journal* **75** (886), 471–474.

Technology Subcommittee of the Working Group on Critical Care (1992) Non-invasive blood gas monitoring: a review for use in the adult critical care unit. *Canadian Medical Association Journal* **146**, 703–712.

Thibodeau, G. & Patton, K. (1999) *Anatomy & Physiology*. Mosby, London.

Torrance, C. & Elley, K. (1997) Respiration, technique and observation 1. *Nursing Times* **43**, suppl.

Trim, J. (2005) Respirations. *Nursing Times* **101** (22), 30–31.

Valenti, L., Tamblyn, R. & Rozinski, M.B. (1997) *Critical Care Nursing*. J B Lippincott, New York.

Wahr, J.A. & Tremper, K.K. (1996) Oxygen measurement and monitoring techniques. In: C. Prys-Roberts & B.R. Brown Jr, eds *International Practice of Anaesthesia*. Butterworth Heinemann, Oxford.

Welch, J. (2005) Pulse oximeters. *Biomedical Instrumentation and Technology* March/April, 125–130.

Welch, J. (1993) Chest drains and pleural drainage. *Surgical Nurse* **6** (5), 7–12.

Weston Smith, S.G.W., Glass, U.H., Acharya, J. *et al.* (1989) Pulse oximetry in sickle cell disease. *Clinical and Laboratory Haematology* **11**, 185–188.

Woodrow, P. (1999) Pulse oximetry. *Nursing Standard* **13** (42), 42–47.

Woodrow, P. (2003) Using non-invasive ventilation in acute ward settings: part 1. *Nursing Standard* **17** (18), 39–44.

Woodrow, P. (2004) Arterial blood gas analysis. *Nursing Standard* **18** (21), 45–52, 54–55.

Woomer, J. & Berkheimer, D. (2003) Using capnography to monitor ventilation. *Nursing* **33** (4), 42–43.

4 | Monitoring Cardiovascular Function 1: ECG Monitoring

INTRODUCTION

ECG monitoring is one of the most valuable diagnostic tools in modern medicine. It is essential if disorders of the cardiac rhythm are to be recognised, and can help with diagnosis and alert healthcare staff to changes in a patient's condition. However ECG monitoring must be meticulously undertaken. Consequences of poor technique include misinterpretation of arrhythmias, mistaken diagnosis, wasted investigations and mismanagement of the patient. Nurses must understand the principles of ECG monitoring, including troubleshooting and recognition of important arrhythmias.

The aim of this chapter is to understand the principles of ECG monitoring.

LEARNING OBJECTIVES

At the end of the chapter the reader will be able to:

❑ describe the common features of a *cardiac monitor*
❑ describe how to set up *ECG monitoring*
❑ discuss the potential *problems* that may be encountered with ECG monitoring
❑ describe the *ECG* and its *relation to cardiac contraction*
❑ describe a systematic approach to *ECG interpretation*
❑ define and classify *cardiac arrhythmias*
❑ *recognise* important cardiac arrhythmias

COMMON FEATURES OF A CARDIAC MONITOR

The bedside cardiac monitor (Fig. 4.1) or oscilloscope provides a continuous display of the patient's ECG and has the following common features:

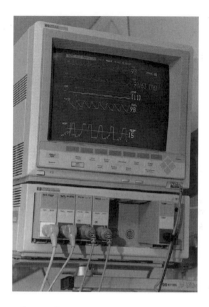

Fig. 4.1 Bedside cardiac monitor.

- *Screen for displaying the ECG trace*: a dull/bright switch can be adjusted if the ECG recording and background is too light or too dark.
- *ECG printout facility*: this is particularly useful for recording cardiac arrhythmias and is invaluable for both diagnostic and treatment purposes. The ECG printouts can also complement the patient's records.
- *Heart rate counter*: most calculate the heart rate by counting the number of QRS complexes in a minute.
- *Monitor alarms*: can alert the nurse to changes in the heart rate that are outside preset limits. If the monitor alarms are to be relied upon, they should be on and set within safe parameters (agreed locally) and based on the patient's clinical condition. More advanced monitors can identify important cardiac arrhythmias and alarm accordingly.
- *Lead select switch*: lead II is usually the most popular lead for ECG monitoring.

- *ECG gain*: this can alter the gain or size of the ECG complex; if it is set too low or too high the ECG trace may be unclear and misinterpreted.
- *Digital processing of the ECG*: potential for electronic analysis.

(Resuscitation Council UK 2006)

SETTING UP ECG MONITORING

The following measures should be observed when setting up ECG monitoring.

1. Explain the procedure to the patient.
2. Prepare the skin: ensure the skin is dry, not greasy; if necessary use an alcohol swab and/or abrasive pad to clean (Resuscitation Council UK 2006). If necessary, shave off any excess hair (Perez 1996a). This will also make it less uncomfortable for the patient when the electrodes are removed.
3. Attach the electrodes following locally agreed guidelines. Switch the cardiac monitor on and select the required monitoring lead.
4. Ensure the ECG trace is clear. Rectify any difficulties encountered (see below).
5. Ensure alarms are set within safe parameters following locally agreed guidelines and according to the patient's clinical condition.
6. Ensure the cardiac monitor can clearly be seen.
7. Document in the patient's notes that ECG monitoring has commenced.

(Adapted from Jevon 2003)

Correct electrode placement (Fig. 4.2) is crucial for obtaining accurate information from any monitoring lead (Jacobson 2000). The electrode placement and monitoring lead selected for ECG monitoring will depend on the factors listed below.

- *Monitoring system* (e.g. three- or five-wire monitoring system). If a five-wire system is being used a suggested ECG electrode placement is red (right shoulder), yellow (left shoulder), green (left lower thorax/hip region), black (right lower thorax/hip region) and white on the chest in the desired V position, usually V1 (Jacobson 2000). If a three-wire system is being used a suggested ECG electrode placement is red (right shoulder), yellow (left shoulder) and green (left lower thorax/hip region).

- *Goals of monitoring*, e.g. if arrhythmia diagnosis is the goal.
- *Patient's clinical situation* (Jacobson 2000): e.g. in cardiopulmonary resuscitation, the precordium should be left unobstructed in case defibrillation is required (Resuscitation Council UK 2006).

EASI 12-lead ECG monitoring

The conventional 12-lead ECG using ten electrodes attached to the limbs and chest is recognised as the current medical standard for the identification, analysis and confirmation of many cardiac abnormalities including cardiac arrhythmias and cardiac ischaemia/infarction.

If 12-lead ECG monitoring is undertaken on a continual basis, the benefits include:

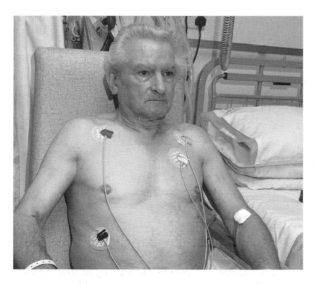

Fig. 4.2 Suggested ECG electrode placement using a five-wire monitoring system.

- Facilitating the accurate recognition of cardiac arrhythmias
- Enabling the monitoring of the mid-precordial leads which is particularly important for the detection and management of ischaemia
- Enabling the recording of *transient* ECG events of particular diagnostic or therapeutic importance
- Enabling the differentiation between post-PTCA (percutaneous transluminal coronary angioplasty) ischaemia and occlusion

Unfortunately the use of a conventional 12-lead ECG system using ten electrodes for continuous cardiac monitoring is cumbersome and generally not practical in the clinical area. However the EASI system, a new concept in 12-lead ECG monitoring, requires the use of only five electrodes (Fig. 4.3):

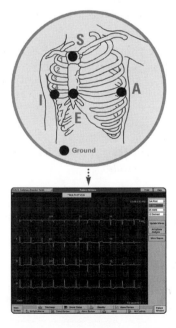

Fig. 4.3 EASI 12-lead ECG monitoring system (reproduced by permission of Philips).

- **E** electrode on the lower sternum at the level of the fifth inter-costal space
- **A** on the left midaxillary line on the same level as the E electrode
- **S** electrode on the upper sternum
- **I** on the right midaxillary line on the same level as the E electrode.

A fifth ground electrode can be placed anywhere.

The EASI system for 12-lead ECG monitoring using only five electrodes is less cumbersome and more practical than the standard ten-electrode system. It is therefore more comfortable for the patient. In addition it will not interfere with such procedures as cardiac auscultation, CPR, defibrillation and echocardiography.

> ECG monitoring should *complement not replace* basic nursing observations of the patient. Treat the patient not the monitor.

POTENTIAL PROBLEMS WITH ECG MONITORING

There are many problems that can occur with ECG monitoring, some are due to the limitations of the monitoring system itself while others are due to poor technique (Meltzer *et al.* 1977). Potential problems that may be encountered include the following.

The 'flat line' trace

Check the patient immediately. However, the most likely cause is mechanical. Check that the:

- correct monitoring lead is selected (usually lead II)
- ECG gain is set correctly
- electrodes are 'in-date' and that the gel sponge is moist, not dry
- electrodes are properly connected
- leads are plugged into the monitor

Poor-quality ECG trace

If the ECG trace quality is poor, check:

- all the connections
- the brightness display

- that the electrodes are 'in-date' and that the gel sponge is moist, not dry (Perez 1996a)
- that the electrodes are properly attached

If there are still difficulties obtaining a clear ECG trace, wiping the skin with an alcohol wipe may help. If the patient is sweating profusely the application of a small amount of tincture benzoin to the skin, leaving it to dry before applying the electrodes, is recommended (Jowett & Thompson 1995). As electrodes tend to dry out after about 3 days, they should be changed at least that often though every 24 hours may be optimum to maintain skin integrity (Perez 1996b).

Interference and artefacts

Poor electrode contact, patient movement and electrical interference, e.g. from bedside infusion pumps, can cause a 'fuzzy' appearance on the ECG trace. Interference can be minimised by applying the electrodes over bone rather than muscle (Resuscitation Council UK 2006). The patient should also be reassured and kept warm.

Wandering baseline

A wandering baseline (ECG trace going up and down) is usually caused by patient movement or simply by respiration. If respiration is the cause and the problem is not transient, repositioning of the electrodes away from the lower ribs is advisable (Meltzer *et al.* 1977).

Small ECG complexes

Sometimes the ECG complexes may be too small and unrecognisable. Possible causes include pericardial effusion, obesity and hypothyroidism. However sometimes it can be caused by a technical problem. Check that the ECG gain is correctly set and lead II is being monitored. Repositioning the electrodes or selecting another monitoring lead sometimes helps.

Incorrect heart rate display

If the ECG complexes are too small, a false low heart rate may be displayed. Large T waves, muscle movement and interference can be mistaken for QRS complexes resulting in a false high heart rate being displayed. The nurse must be alert to the possibility of inaccurate heart rate readings, which can in particular be caused by poor electrode contact and interference (Ren *et al.* 1998). To minimise the potential for inaccuracies, a reliable good-quality ECG trace should be obtained.

Skin irritation

ECG electrodes can cause skin irritation. The electrode sites should be regularly examined and if the patient's skin appears irritated select another electrode placement (Paul & Hebra 1998).

False alarms

Frequent false alarms will undermine the rationale for setting alarms and can also cause undue anxiety for the patient. It is important to ensure that the alarms are correctly and sensibly set and that the ECG is accurate, reliable and of a high standard.

Best practice – ECG monitoring

Ensure adequate skin preparation
Use ECG electrodes that are in date, with moist gel sponge
Position ECG electrodes and select monitoring lead following locally
  agreed protocols
Set cardiac monitor alarms according to the patient's clinical
  condition
Ensure the ECG trace is accurate
Ensure the cardiac monitor is visible

THE ECG AND ITS RELATION TO CARDIAC CONTRACTION

The ECG functions in four stages as follows (Fig. 4.4):

1. The sinus node fires and the electrical impulse spreads across the atria. This results in atrial contraction (P wave).
2. On arriving at the AV junction the impulse is delayed, allowing the atria time to contract fully and eject blood into the ventricles. This brief period of absent electrical activity is

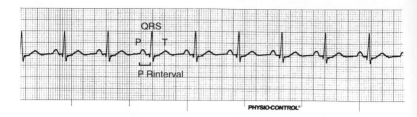

Fig. 4.4 The ECG and its relation to cardiac contraction (PQRST complex).

represented on the ECG by a straight (isoelectric) line between the end of the P wave and the beginning of the QRS complex. The PR interval represents atrial depolarisation and the impulse delay in the AV junction prior to ventricular depolarisation.

3. The impulse is then conducted down to the ventricles through the bundle of His, right and left bundle branches and Purkinje fibres, causing ventricular depolarisation and contraction (QRS complex).

4. The ventricles then repolarise (T wave).

SYSTEMATIC APPROACH TO ECG INTERPRETATION

It is important to develop a systematic approach to ECG interpretation and to apply it consistently: this will minimise the risk of missing something important (Aehlert 2006).

The following systematic approach to ECG interpretation enables the practitioner to interpret most ECG traces and arrive at a reliable diagnosis on which to base effective treatment. The six-stage approach is as follows:

- Electrical activity: present?
- QRS rate: normal, slow or fast?
- QRS rhythm: regular or irregular?
- QRS width: normal or wide?
- P waves: present?
- P waves and QRS: associated or disassociated?

(Resuscitation Council UK 2006)

Electrical activity

If there is no electrical activity present, assuming the patient has a pulse, check that the leads and electrodes are correctly attached, check that the ECG gain is not too low and that the correct monitoring lead has been selected, e.g. lead II. If electrical activity is present and recognisable QRS complexes can be seen, proceed to checking the QRS rate, QRS rhythm, QRS width, P waves and the relationship between P waves and QRS complexes (Resuscitation Council UK 2006).

QRS rate

Estimate the QRS rate by counting the number of large (1 cm) squares between adjacent QRS complexes and dividing it into 300, e.g. the QRS rate in Fig. 4.4 is approximately 80/min (300/3.8) (Perez 1996a).

- Normal ventricular rate is 60–100 beats/min.
- Bradycardia – rate <60 beats/min.
- Tachycardia – rate >100 beats/min.

(Leach, 2004)

If the QRS rhythm is irregular it is preferable to estimate the rate by counting the number of QRS complexes in a 15-second ECG strip and then multiplying it by four.

QRS rhythm

Determine whether the QRS rhythm is regular or irregular. It is important to assess the regularity of the QRS rhythm using an adequate length of ECG rhythm strip (Resuscitation Council UK 2006). Compare R–R intervals by either using a calliper or by marking two consecutive R waves on a piece of paper and then comparing the marks with other R–R intervals on the ECG rhythm strip.

If it is irregular, establish if there is a common pattern or whether it is very erratic. Causes of an irregular QRS rhythm include sinus arrhythmia, premature complexes and some atrioventricular (AV) blocks. If the QRS rhythm is very erratic, it is most likely to be atrial fibrillation, particularly if the QRS width is normal (Resuscitation Council UK 2006).

QRS width

Calculate the QRS width. The upper limit of normal is 0.12 seconds or 3 small squares (Resuscitation Council UK 2006). Causes of a wide QRS complex include bundle branch block, ventricular premature contractions and ventricular tachycardia.

P waves

Determine whether P waves are present. They should be upright in lead II and be all of the same morphology. P waves of different morphology indicate a changing atrial pacemaker. P waves may be absent in some conduction disturbances and sometimes they may be difficult to distinguish or indeed be 'hidden' in the QRS in some tachyarrhythmias.

Relationship between the P waves and the QRS complexes

If P waves are present, establish whether a P wave precedes each QRS complex and that each QRS complex is followed by a P wave. Calculate the PR interval: it should remain constant and the normal range is 3–5 small squares. A shortened or prolonged PR interval is indicative of a conduction abnormality. A prolonged PR interval can be seen in AV block. Complete dissociation between the P waves and QRS complexes is most commonly seen in third-degree or complete AV heart block.

Sinus rhythm

This is illustrated in Fig. 1.3.

QRS rate: 80/min
QRS rhythm: regular
P waves: present and normal
Relationship between P waves and QRS: the P waves precede each QRS and the PR interval is normal
QRS width: normal (<2.5 squares)

The impulse originates in the sinus node at a rate of between 60 and 100 beats/min, is regular and is conducted down the normal pathways and with no abnormal delays, i.e. sinus rhythm.

> **Best practice – ECG interpretation**
>
> Assess the patient for adverse signs
> Calculate the QRS rate
> Ascertain the QRS rhythm
> Identify if P waves are present
> Assess the relationship between P waves and QRS complexes
> Calculate the QRS width
> Obtain 12-lead ECG if necessary

DEFINITION AND CLASSIFICATION OF CARDIAC ARRHYTHMIAS

A 'cardiac arrhythmia' can be defined as any ECG rhythm that deviates from normal sinus rhythm. Cardiac arrhythmias can be classified into one of two groups (Meltzer *et al.* 1977):

- arrhythmias resulting from a disturbance in impulse *formation*
- arrhythmias resulting from a disturbance in impulse *conduction*

> Some cardiac arrhythmias may have a disturbance in both impulse formation and impulse conduction.

Arrhythmias resulting from a disturbance in impulse formation

These arrhythmias can be classified in respect of their site of origin and the mechanism of the disturbance as shown below (adapted from Jevon 2000).

Site of origin

The following features are significant:

- *SA node*: sinus rhythms, e.g. sinus bradycardia, sinus tachycardia
- *atria*: atrial rhythms, e.g. atrial premature, atrial fibrillation
- *AV junction*: junctional rhythms, e.g. junction rhythm
- *ventricles*: ventricular rhythms, e.g. ventricular premature beats, ventricular tachycardia

Mechanism

Features arising from the mechanism of the disturbance are:

- tachycardia >100 beats/minute
- bradycardia <60 beats/minute
- premature contractions
- flutter
- fibrillation

Arrhythmias resulting from a disturbance in impulse conduction

A disturbance in conduction relates to an abnormal delay or block of the impulse at any point along the conduction system. They are traditionally categorised according to the site of the defect:

- *sinoatrial blocks*, e.g. sinus arrest
- *atrioventricular blocks*, e.g. first-, second-, third-degree block
- *intraventricular blocks*, e.g. right and left bundle branch blocks

RECOGNITION OF IMPORTANT ARRHYTHMIAS

When interpreting arrhythmias it is important to assess:

- the haemodynamic effect: clinical signs of a low cardiac output include hypotension, impaired consciousness, chest pain, dyspnoea and heart failure (European Resuscitation Council 1998)
- whether there is a risk of cardiac arrest

Sinus tachycardia

This is illustrated in Fig. 4.5.

Electrical activity and recognisable QRS complexes: present
QRS rate: 120/min
QRS rhythm: regular
QRS width: normal
P waves: present and normal
Relationship between P waves and QRS complexes: P waves precede every QRS complex; PR interval normal

The ECG shows the same characteristics as sinus rhythm except that the ventricular (QRS) rate is >100 beats/min. Causes include anxiety, acute blood loss, exercise, shock, pyrexia and drugs, e.g.

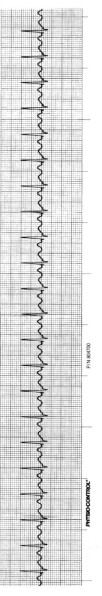

Fig. 4.5 Sinus tachycardia.

hydralazine, nebulised salbutamol. Of greater importance is that it may be a manifestation of heart failure when it is a reflex mechanism to compensate for reduced stroke volume (Meltzer *et al.* 1977). The treatment is to identify and treat the cause (Leach 2004). Sometimes beta blockers are beneficial, e.g. in acute myocardial infarction.

Sinus bradycardia
Sinus brachycardia is illustrated in Fig. 4.6.

Electrical activity and recognisable QRS complexes: present
QRS rate: 40/min
QRS rhythm: regular
QRS width: normal
P waves: present and normal
Relationship between P waves and QRS complexes: P waves precede
    each QRS complex and the PR interval is normal

ECG shows the same characteristics as sinus rhythm except that the ventricular rate is <60 beats/min. Causes include vagal stimulation, e.g. during tracheal suction, increased intracranial pressure, hypoxia, severe pain, hypothermia and drugs, e.g. beta blockers. Sometimes it is normal for the patient, e.g. an athlete. Treatment often requires oxygen and atropine. Sometimes pacing may be indicated. The treatment required will depend on the risk of developing asystole, rather than the precise classification of the bradycardia (Resuscitation Council UK 2006).

Atrial fibrillation
This is illustrated in Fig. 4.7.

Electrical activity and recognisable QRS complexes: present
QRS rate: 140/min
QRS rhythm: irregular and very erratic
QRS width: normal
P waves: not present, irregular baseline – small, irregular and
    rapid oscillations
Relationship between P waves and QRS complexes: no P waves
    present

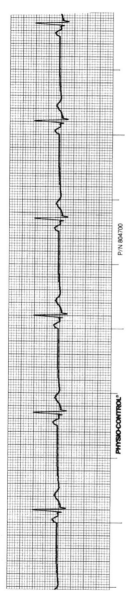

Fig. 4.6 Sinus bradycardia.

PHYSIO-CONTROL®

P/N 804700

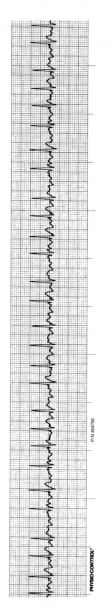

Fig. 4.7 Atrial fibrillation.

Atrial fibrillation is characterised by absent P waves, irregular baseline and irregular QRS complexes. The loss of atrial contraction or 'atrial kick' results in a 25% reduction in cardiac output. It is the most common cardiac arrhythmia encountered in clinical practice (Resuscitation Council UK 2006). The ventricular rate can vary and treatment often includes digoxin. Cardioversion is sometimes required.

Atrial flutter

Atrial flutter is illustrated in Fig. 4.8.

Electrical activity and recognisable QRS complexes: present
QRS rate: 100/min
QRS rhythm: regular
QRS width: normal
P waves: flutter 'sawtooth' waves at a rate of 300/minute
Relationship between P waves and QRS complexes: has no meaning and is not measured

Atrial flutter is characterised by the 'sawtooth' flutter waves which usually have a rate of approximately 300/minute. The ventricular response depends on the degree of atrioventricular block; in the example it is 3:1. Treatment could include digoxin or amiodarone. Cardioversion may be required.

Narrow complex tachycardia

The features of this are shown in Fig. 4.9.

Electrical activity and recognisable QRS complexes: present
QRS rate: 180/min

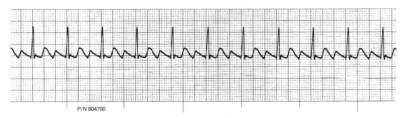

P/N 804700

Fig. 4.8 Atrial flutter.

103

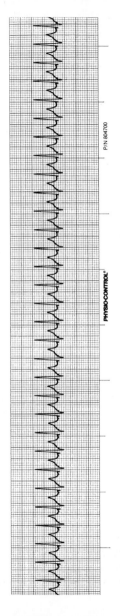

Fig. 4.9 Narrow complex tachycardia.

QRS rhythm: regular
QRS width: normal
P waves: unable to identify (situated on T waves?)
Relationship between P waves and QRS complexes: unable to
determine

Unlike sinus tachycardia, narrow complex tachycardia (sometimes referred to as supraventricular tachycardia) starts and ends
abruptly. The rate is always >140 beats/minute. A 12-lead ECG
will help to determine the exact diagnosis. The key issue with this
ECG is the QRS width, which rules out the often more serious
broad complex (ventricular) tachycardia. Treatment, which will
depend on how compromised the patient is, could include vagal
manoeuvres, adenosine, amiodarone and cardioversion.

Broad complex tachycardia

Fig. 4.10 shows the salient features of broad complex tachycardia.

Electrical activity and recognisable QRS complexes: present
QRS rate: 180/min
QRS rhythm: regular
P waves: not seen
Relationship between P waves and QRS complexes: unable to
determine
QRS width: wide

Broad complex tachycardia usually results from a focus in the
ventricles firing at a rapid rate. The patient may or may not lose
cardiac output. The ECG shows a rapid heart rate usually over
150/minute and the QRS complex is characteristically wide (more
than 3 small squares). The ECG configuration can vary depending
on where in the ventricles the focus is. If the patient has
arrested the definitive treatment is rapid defibrillation. Other
treatment could include drugs, e.g. lignocaine or amiodarone,
and cardioversion.

Ventricular fibrillation

In ventricular fibrillation all coordination of electrical activity in
the ventricular myocardium is lost, resulting in cardiac arrest.
The ECG is characteristic, a bizarre irregular waveform apparently

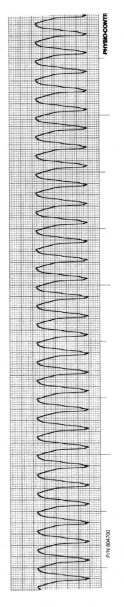

Fig. 4.10 Broad complex tachycardia.

random in both frequency and amplitude. It can be classified as either coarse (Fig. 1.1) or fine (Fig. 4.11). Certainly the latter is significant in resuscitation because it can be mistaken for asystole, particularly if there is some interference. The definitive treatment is rapid defibrillation (Resuscitation Council UK 2006).

Asystole

Asystole (Fig. 1.2) is characteristically an undulating line and rarely a straight line.

In all cases of apparent asystole, the ECG trace should be viewed with suspicion before arrival at a final diagnosis. Check the patient. Other causes of a straight line ECG trace should be excluded, e.g. incorrect lead setting, disconnected leads and ECG gain incorrectly set. It is important not to miss ventricular fibrillation.

Pulseless electrical activity

Pulseless electrical activity (see Fig. 1.3) is a condition in which the patient is pulseless, but has a normal ECG trace. The diagnosis is made from a combination of the clinical absence of a cardiac output together with an ECG trace that would normally be associated with a good pulse.

Scenario

A 40-year-old man is admitted to the Coronary Care Unit with an acute inferior myocardial infarction. On admission BP is 120/90, pulse 70/minute, sinus rhythm, resps 15/minute and temperature 36.7°C. The cardiac monitor starts to alarm as it has recognised 'asystole'. What would you do?

First of all check the patient. He is conscious, sitting up in bed and smiling. The cardiac monitor is still alarming 'asystole'. What would you do?

The ECG display is a straight line, which the monitor has mistaken for asystole. There must be a mechanical problem. The lead select on the cardiac monitor is checked to ensure the desired lead has been selected. In addition the ECG gain (size) on the monitor is checked and is found to be fine. The leads are checked to ensure they are still connected. One of the leads has become disconnected from the electrode resulting in a straight line on the ECG. Following reconnection, sinus rhythm 70 BPM is displayed on the cardiac monitor.

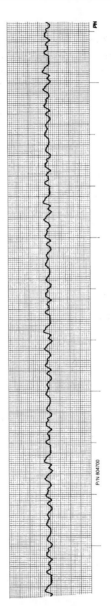

Fig. 4.11 Ventricular fibrillation (fine).

CONCLUSION

ECG monitoring is central to the care of a critically ill patient. It must be meticulously undertaken in order to avoid misinterpretation of arrhythmias, mistaken diagnosis, wasted investigations and mismanagement of the patient. Nurses need to understand the principles of ECG monitoring, including troubleshooting, and recognise important cardiac arrhythmias. Always remember to treat the patient not the monitor.

REFERENCES

Aehlert, B. (2006) *Pocket Reference for ECGs Made Easy* 3rd edn. Mosby, Elsevier, Missouri.

European Resuscitation Council (1998) *European Resuscitation Council Guidelines for Resuscitation*. Elsevier, Oxford.

Jacobson, C. (2000) Optimum bedside cardiac monitoring. *Progress in Cardiovascular Nursing* **15** (4), 134–137.

Jevon, P. (2000) Cardiac monitoring. *Nursing Times* **96** (23), 43.

Jevon, P. (2003) *ECGs for Nurses*. Blackwell Publishing, Oxford.

Jowett, N.I. & Thompson, D.R. (1995) *Comprehensive Coronary Care* 2nd edn. Scutari Press/RCN, London.

Leach, R. (2004) *Critical Care Medicine at a Glance*. Blackwell Publishing, Oxford.

Meltzer, L.E., Pinneo, R. & Kitchell, J.R. (1977) *Intensive Coronary Care, a Manual for Nurses* 3rd edn. Prentice-Hall, London.

Paul, S. & Hebra, J. (1998) *The Nurse's Guide to Cardiac Rhythm Interpretation*. W.B. Saunders. Philadelphia.

Perez, A. (1996a) Cardiac monitoring: mastering the essentials. *Registered Nurse* **59** (8), 32–39.

Perez, A. (1996b) ECG electrode placement: a refresher course. *Registered Nurse* **59** (9), 29–31.

Ren, Y., Yang, L. & Hu, P. (1998) Analysis of influencing factors on ECG monitoring. *Shanxi Nursing Journal* **12** (5), 213–214.

Resuscitation Council UK (2006) *Advanced Life Support* 5th edn. Resuscitation Council UK, London.

5 | Monitoring Cardiovascular Function 2: Haemodynamic Monitoring

INTRODUCTION

Haemodynamics can be defined as the study of the physical aspects of blood circulation, including cardiac function and peripheral vascular physiological characteristics (Mosby 1998). Haemodynamic monitoring is central to the care of a critically ill patient and can be classified as *non-invasive, invasive* and *derived* (i.e. data calculated from other measurements).

'Haemodynamic measurements are important to establish a precise diagnosis, determine appropriate therapy and monitor the response to that therapy' (Gomersall & Oh 1997). In particular they can assist in the early recognition of shock, where the immediate provision of circulatory support is paramount (Hinds & Watson 1999).

The aim of this chapter is to understand the principles of haemodynamic monitoring.

LEARNING OBJECTIVES

At the end of the chapter the reader will be able to:

❏ discuss the factors affecting *tissue perfusion*
❏ define and classify *circulatory shock*
❏ describe non-invasive methods of *haemodynamic monitoring*
❏ outline the general principles of monitoring with *transducers*
❏ discuss the principles of *central venous pressure monitoring*
❏ outline and discuss the principles of *pulmonary artery pressure monitoring*
❏ discuss the principles of *cardiac output studies*

FACTORS AFFECTING TISSUE PERFUSION

Tissue perfusion is dependent upon an adequate blood pressure in the aorta. This pressure is determined by the product of two factors: *cardiac output* and *peripheral resistance* (Green 1991) (Fig. 5.1).

Cardiac output

Cardiac output is the amount of blood ejected from the left ventricle in 1 minute. At rest this is approximately 5000 ml. It is determined by heart rate and stroke volume.

Heart rate

Factors influencing heart rate include baroreceptor activity, the Bainbridge effect, pyrexia, higher centres, intracranial pressure and oxygen and carbon dioxide levels in the blood.

Stroke volume

Stroke volume is the amount of blood ejected from the left ventricle in one contraction. At rest this is approximately 70 ml. It is affected by heart rate, myocardial contractility, preload and afterload (Fig. 5.1).

- *Heart rate*: tachycardia reduces diastolic filling time resulting in a decreased stroke volume.
- *Myocardial contractility* refers to the ability of the heart to function independently of the changes in preload and afterload (Hinds & Watson 1996). It is commonly referred to as the 'force of contraction'. Inotropic drugs, e.g. dobutamine, adrenaline, can increase myocardial contractility. Table 5.1 lists factors affecting myocardial contractility.

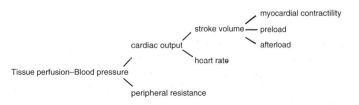

Fig. 5.1 Overview of factors affecting tissue perfusion.

Table 5.1 Factors affecting myocardial contractility.

Change	Factors
Increased contractility	Drugs with inotropic properties, e.g. dobutamine, dopamine (dose related), digoxin, adrenaline, noradrenaline; circulating catecholamines; calcium; increased preload; hyperthyroidism
Decreased contractility	Drugs with negative inotropic properties, e.g. lignocaine; hypoxia; hypocalcaemia and calcium channel blockers; beta adrenergic blockers, e.g. atenolol; decreased preload; functional deficit, e.g. following myocardial infarction

Table 5.2 Factors affecting preload.

Change	Factors
Increased preload	Volume gain, e.g. fluid overload; renal failure; vasoconstriction (may be caused by drugs, e.g. noradrenaline, adrenaline and dopamine (dose related)); heart failure; hypothermia and anxiety; bradycardia
Decreased preload	Volume loss, e.g. haemorrhage, severe vomiting and polyuria; vasodilatation, e.g. anaphylaxis, septicaemia, pyrexia, neurogenic shock and drugs such as nitrates; impeded venous return, e.g. pulmonary embolism, pericardial tamponade; tachycardia (fall in diastolic filling time)

- *Preload* (or end diastolic volume/pressure) is the tension of the myocardial fibres at the end of diastole just before ventricular contraction (Hinds & Watson 1996). Starling's law of the heart states that 'the force of myocardial contraction is directly proportional to the initial fibre length', i.e. stretched fibres contract more forcefully (not overstretched). Venous return is the main factor determining preload and as the filling pressure rises, stroke volume increases. However in an overstretched ventricle, excessive dilatation may result in a fall in stroke volume. In the clinical setting manipulation of the preload is the most efficient method of improving cardiac output because it is associated with only a minimal rise in oxygen consumption (Hinds & Watson 1996). Table 5.2 lists factors affecting preload.

• *Afterload* is the resistance to the outflow of blood provided by the vasculature which must be overcome by the ventricles during contraction. In the clinical setting a rise in afterload, particularly in the failing heart, results in a decrease in cardiac output (Lee & Branch 1997). Table 5.3 lists factors affecting afterload.

Peripheral resistance

Peripheral resistance is the resistance to the flow of blood determined by the tone of the vascular musculature and the diameter of the blood vessels (Mosby 1998).

The smooth muscle in the arterioles is controlled by the vasomotor centre in the medulla. It is in a state of partial contraction caused by continuous sympathetic nerve activity, often referred to as 'sympathetic tone'. An increase in vasomotor activity causes vasoconstriction of the arterioles resulting in a rise in peripheral resistance. If the cardiac output remains constant the blood pressure will rise. In contrast, a decrease in vasomotor activity causes vasodilation and a fall in peripheral resistance. If the cardiac output remains constant the blood pressure will fall. The most significant factors affecting vasomotor activity are listed below:

• *Baroreceptor activity* helps to maintain the blood pressure at a constant level. Baroreceptors are located in the aortic arch, carotid arteries and carotid sinus. Baroreceptor activity inhibits the action of the vasomotor centre: a rise in blood pressure increases, and a fall decreases, baroreceptor activity. When moving from a lying to a standing position, the cardiac output will fall. However baroreceptor activity ensures that the blood pressure remains constant. Following prolonged bed rest this mechanism may be lost and the patient may faint.

Table 5.3 Factors affecting afterload.

Change	Factors
Increased afterload	Drugs with vasoconstriction properties, e.g. noradrenaline; cardiogenic shock; atherosclerosis
Decreased afterload	Drugs with vasodilator properties, e.g. nitrates, nitroprusside; anaphylaxsis; septicaemia; hyperthermia

- *Carbon dioxide (CO_2)*: a rise in blood carbon dioxide levels increases vasomotor activity, whilst a fall suppresses it. In ventilated patients care needs to be taken to avoid over-ventilation as this may lead to a fall in carbon dioxide levels with a corresponding fall in blood pressure.
- *Sensory nerves* can influence vasomotor activity, particularly those which are associated with pain. Mild pain can increase vasomotor activity resulting in a rise in blood pressure, whilst severe pain may decrease vasomotor activity and cause a fall in blood pressure.
- *Respiratory centre*: this lies next to the vasomotor centre; an increase in its activity, particularly on inspiration, will result in an increase in vasomotor activity causing a rise in blood pressure.
- *Oxygen (O_2)*: a moderate fall in blood oxygen levels increases vasomotor activity directly and also indirectly via chemoreceptors.
- *Higher centres*: emotional excitement or stress results in a rise in vasomotor activity and a corresponding rise in blood pressure. In some situations inhibition of the vasomotor centre will occur resulting in vasodilation and a fall in blood pressure, for instance, some people faint at the sight of blood.

There are other factors that affect peripheral resistance including:

- *Angiotensin*: inadequate renal blood flow leads to the release of the enzyme renin which causes the formation of angiotensin, a powerful vasoconstrictor.
- *Blood viscosity*: if the blood viscosity increases, e.g. in polycythaemia, peripheral resistance will also rise.
- *Stimulation of alpha and beta 2 receptors* (found in the smooth muscle of the arterioles): stimulation of alpha receptors, e.g. by noradrenaline, will cause vasoconstriction; stimulation of beta 2 receptors, e.g. by salbutamol, will cause vasodilation.

CLASSIFICATION OF CIRCULATORY SHOCK
Circulatory shock can be defined as acute circulatory failure with inadequate or inappropriately distributed tissue perfusion resulting in generalised cellular hypoxia (Graham & Parke

2005). A complex physiological phenomenon, shock is a life-threatening condition with a variety of causes. Without treatment it leads to cell starvation, cell death, organ dysfunction, organ failure and eventually death (Collins 2000; Hand 2001). The presence of shock is best detected by looking for signs of compromised end organ perfusion (Graham & Parke 2005).

Haemodynamic monitoring will assist nurses in recognising the early signs of shock, facilitate timely management, evaluate treatment response and potentially reverse the early stages of deadly sequelae.

The prognosis of shock will depend upon the underlying cause, severity and duration of the shocked state. The patient's age and pre-existing illness (co-morbidity) are also contributing factors. There are four major classifications of shock: cardiogenic, hypovolaemic, distributive and obstructive (Bridges & Dukes 2005).

Hypovolaemic shock

Although the heart may be pumping effectively, loss of circulating volume results in a low perfusion state (Collins 2000) and reduced oxygen delivery. Causes of hypovolaemia are either from internal fluid shifts or external fluid losses (Diehl-Oplinger & Kaminski 2004). Fluid shifts from intravascular compartments to 'third spaces' (intracellular or extracellular compartments), which do not support the circulation, can be the result of intestinal obstruction, vomiting and diarrhoea, pancreatitis, peritonitis, burns and excessive diuretic therapy (Collins 2000; Diehl-Oplinger & Kaminski 2004). External fluid loss can be caused by haemorrhage, severe vomiting, osmotic diuresis, trauma and surgery (Hand 2001).

Cardiogenic shock

Cardiogenic shock is caused by severe heart failure (Leach 2004) usually secondary to acute myocardial infarction (AMI) but can also follow cardiomyopathy, trauma or myocarditis (Collins 2000). Because of a reduced cardiac output, catecholamines (adrenaline and noradrenaline), renin and aldosterone are released, which cause a tachycardia and vasoconstriction, increasing afterload, myocardial workload and oxygen consumption. Haemodynamic readings will demonstrate tachycardia, falling systolic blood pressure, low cardiac output, high pulmonary artery wedge pressure, increased systemic vascular resistance (SVR) and a fall in left ventricular stroke volume (LVSV) (Green 1991).

Distributive shock

Distributive shock arises from abnormality of the peripheral circulation and can be divided into three different types: neurogenic, anaphylactic and septic (Hand 2001). Despite an adequate circulating volume, the vasculature expands until it can no longer maintain the pressure within it (Hand 2001); venous return will fall leading to a fall in cardiac output.

Although cardiac output could rise, the uptake of oxygen is impaired; there is still a relative low volume because the intravascular space has increased due to the dilation of the systemic vasculature. In sepsis and anaphylaxis capillaries become permeable because of circulating inflammatory mediators. This permeability causes fluid leakage from the vasculature to the interstitial space, further reducing intravascular volume. Neurogenic shock can be caused by damage to the spinal cord or brainstem, emotional trauma or drugs which cause a reduction of sympathetic impulses causing massive vasodilation (Collins 2000).

Haemodynamic readings initially appear normal or show an increase in cardiac output, fall in SVR and low to normal pulmonary artery wedge pressure (PAWP) as a hyperdynamic state develops to compensate for reducing cardiac output.

Obstructive shock

Obstructive shock is caused by circulatory obstruction (Leach 2004). Causes include pulmonary embolism, tension pneumothorax and cardiac tamponade.

Haemodynamic readings show a fall in cardiac output, fall in PAWP and a rise in SVR. Pressures in the right side of the heart, pulmonary artery and left chambers equilibrate in diastole, while cardiac output falls, SVR rises and PAWP is variable dependent on the cause of the obstruction.

NON-INVASIVE METHODS OF HAEMODYNAMIC MONITORING

This section discusses the various non-invasive methods of haemodynamic monitoring. A non-invasive monitoring device is illustrated in Fig. 5.2.

Assessment of respiratory rate

Respiratory rate is an early significant indicator of cellular dysfunction. This is a sensitive physiological indicator and should be monitored and recorded regularly. Rate and depth of respirations will initially increase in response to cellular hypoxia.

Assessment of pulse and ECG

A rapid, weak, thready pulse is a characteristic sign of shock (Collins 2000). A full bounding or throbbing pulse may be indicative of anaemia, heart block, heart failure or the early stages of septic shock; the hyperdynamic or compensatory stage. A

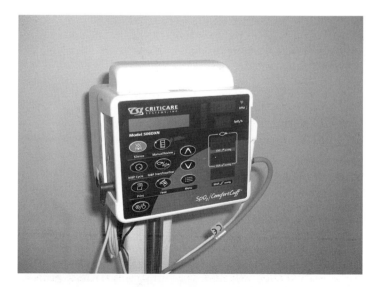

Fig. 5.2 Non-invasive blood pressure monitoring device.

discrepancy in the volume between central and distal pulses may be caused by a fall in cardiac output (and also cold ambient temperature).

ECG monitoring is an invaluable non-invasive method of continuous monitoring of the heart rate. It can provide the practitioner with an early sign of a fall in cardiac output. The principles of ECG monitoring have been discussed in Chapter 4.

Assessment of cerebral perfusion

Altered mental state (Robson & Newell 2005), such as a deterioration in conscious level, confusion, agitation and lethargy, is an important determinant of cerebral perfusion and the presence of shock.

Assessment of skin perfusion

Decreased skin perfusion is often characterised by cool peripheries, skin mottling, pallor, cyanosis and delayed capillary refill time (CRT). The following procedure is suggested for the assessment of CRT:

- Explain the procedure to the patient.
- Elevate the digit to the level of the heart (or slightly higher). This will ensure the assessment of arteriolar capillary and not venous stasis refill.
- Apply sufficient pressure to cause blanching to the digit for 5 seconds and then release (Resuscitation Council UK 2006).
- Time how long it takes for the colour of the skin to return to the same colour of the surrounding tissues, i.e. capillary refill time. The normal CRT is <2 seconds (Gwinnutt 2006).

A sluggish (delayed) CRT (>2 seconds) suggests poor peripheral perfusion. Other factors that can prolong CRT include a cold ambient temperature, poor lighting and old age (Resuscitation Council UK 2006).

Assessment of urine output

Urine output can indirectly provide an indication of cardiac output. In health 25% of the cardiac output perfuses the kidneys. When renal perfusion is adequate, urine output should exceed 0.5 ml/kg per hour (Gomersall & Oh 1997). Decreased urine output may be an early sign of hypovolaemia because when cardiac output falls so does renal perfusion (Druding 2000). Once urine output is less than approximately 500 ml/day, the kidneys are unable to excrete the waste products of metabolism; uraemia, metabolic acidosis and hyperkalaemia will develop (Gwinnutt 2006).

In the critically ill patient, acute renal failure is usually caused by inadequate renal perfusion pressure (pre-renal failure) caused by, for example, hypovolaemia (Gwinnutt 2006). If diuretics have been administered, e.g. frusemide urine output is not helpful in assessing cardiac output (Duke *et al*. 1994). If the patient is catheterised, ensure that the tube is not blocked or kinked.

Arterial blood pressure measurements

Arterial blood pressure (ABP) is the force exerted by the circulating volume of blood on the walls of the arteries (Mosby 1998). Changes in cardiac output or peripheral resistance can affect the blood pressure. A patient with a low cardiac output can maintain a normal blood pressure by vasoconstriction, whilst a patient who is vasodilated may be hypotensive despite a high cardiac output, e.g. in sepsis. Mean arterial pressure (MAP) is an average pressure reading within the arterial system (Garretson 2005) and is a useful indicator as it can approximate perfusion to essential organs such as the kidneys. MAP is recognised as the main therapeutic endpoint for a patient with sepsis (Giuliano 2006).

'The adequacy of blood pressure in an individual patient must always be assessed in relation to their premorbid value' (Hinds & Watson 1996). Table 5.4 provides an indication of 'expected' systolic and diastolic blood pressure measurements. Hypotension can lead to inadequate perfusion of vital organs. Hypertension increases myocardial workload and can precipitate cerebral vascular accidents.

Cardiac output is related to pulse pressure, which is the difference between the systolic and diastolic pressures, usually 30–40 mmHg (Mosby 1998). Following a fall in cardiac output the pulse pressure will narrow, resulting in a thready pulse. In the early stages of septic shock, the cardiac output can rise, resulting in a wide pulse pressure and bounding pulses.

Table 5.4 Normal intracardiac pressures.

Parameter	Normal range
Central venous	0 to +8 mmHg (right atrial level)
Right ventricle	0 to +8 mmHg diastolic +15 to +30 mmHg systolic
Pulmonary capillary wedge pressure	+5 to +15 mmHg
Left atrium	+4 to +12 mmHg
Left ventricle	+4 to +12 mmHg diastolic +90 to +140 mmHg systolic
Aorta	+90 to +140 mmHg systolic +60 to +90 mmHg diastolic +70 to +105 mmHg mean

Reproduced with kind permission of Routledge from Woodrow P. (2000) *Intensive Care Nursing*, p. 212.

Factors influencing blood pressure measurements

There are numerous factors that can influence blood pressure, e.g. nicotine, anxiety, pain, position of patient, medications, exercise. It is important to ensure a standardised approach is used to minimise the impact of extraneous variables on blood pressure (Torrance & Semple 1997).

Although the blood pressure reading in the left arm is generally a more accurate reflection of arterial blood pressure (Torrance & Semple 1997), blood pressure measurement should be recorded in the arm with the highest reading (O'Brien *et al.* 1995). Wide discrepancies between right and left arm blood pressure measurements may be indicative of an aortic aneurysm.

Factors affecting accuracy of blood pressure measurements

The accuracy of blood pressure measurement may be affected by the following factors:

- *Cuff width*: if this is too narrow the blood pressure reading will be falsely high while if it is too wide it will be falsely low (British Hypertension Society 2006). The European Standard recommends that the width of the bladder should be 40%, and the length 80–100%, of the limb circumference (CEN 1995; British Hypertension Society 2006).

- *Position of the arm*: the arm should be supported in a horizontal position at the level of the heart. Incorrect positioning during the procedure can lead to errors of as much as 10% (O'Brien *et al.* 1995).

Complications

Complications associated with non-invasive blood pressure devices include limb oedema, friction blisters and ulnar nerve palsy if the cuff is placed too low on the upper arm (British Hypertension Society 2006). If the patient is being thrombolysed, e.g. following myocardial infarction, over-inflation or frequent inflations could cause excessive bruising (Smith 2000).

GENERAL PRINCIPLES OF MONITORING WITH TRANSDUCERS

Transducers enable the pressure readings from invasive monitoring of the patient to be displayed on a monitor, i.e. arterial lines or central venous pressure (CVP) lines. To maintain patency of the cannula and tubing and prevent back-flow of blood, a bag of normal saline should be connected to the transducer tubing and kept under continuous pressure of 300 mmHg (i.e. greater than arterial pressure), thus facilitating a continuous flush at 3 ml/hour.

Best practice – monitoring with transducers

Check flush bag each shift – if it runs too low the line will clot off
Ensure the pressure bag remains inflated at 300 mmHg – to ensure continuous flushing
If flat trace check for breaks in the circuit and air – rectify safely and flush line
If trace remains flat withdraw blood while manipulating limb
Always check the patient – asystole causes a flat trace

Ensuring accuracy

The following precautions will help to ensure accuracy of measurements:

- Keep the transducer level with the zero reference point, usually the mid-axilla. Always use the same reference point in order to ensure meaningful comparison.
- Limit the use of three-way taps.
- Remove any air bubbles from the system.
- Calibrate the transducer to atmospheric pressure prior to and regularly during use. This should be undertaken following the manufacturer's recommendations and is typically as follows:
  1. Switch the three-way tap in the tubing open to air (atmospheric pressure) and off to the patient.
  2. Press the zero button on the monitor and observe for 0 to be displayed.
  3. Switch the three-way tap off to air and open to the patient.
  4. Ensure that the transducer is at the zero reference point and observe for the pressure trace on the monitor.

Principles of arterial pressure monitoring

Indications for insertion of an arterial line include the requirement for continuous monitoring of arterial blood pressure in critically ill patients (Garretson 2005), when using potent vasoactive drugs such as adrenaline and noradrenaline, and frequent blood sampling, e.g. blood gas and acid–base analysis.

Best practice – monitoring an arterial line

Ensure arterial line is clearly labelled 'arterial'

Limb should be exposed and constantly observed for signs of a decrease in perfusion and disconnection of the cannula (Garretson 2005)

Use transparent dressing so site can be monitored for signs of infection

Ensure monitor alarms are set following local protocols

If flat trace observed, once asystole excluded, identify and rectify cause of problem

---

Common insertion sites

The radial artery (alternative sites include the brachial, dorsalis pedis and femoral arteries) is usually the site of choice; advantages include:

- superficial position
- readily accessible
- easy to monitor and observe
- easy to apply pressure in the event of bleeding
- minimal restriction to patient movement
- adequate collateral circulation is normally present (Hinds & Watson 1999)

The arterial waveform

The arterial waveform reflects the pressure generated in the arteries following ventricular contraction and should correlate with the QRS of the ECG (Garretson 2005). Figure 5.3 depicts a typical arterial waveform and its configuration can be described as follows:

- *Anacrotic notch*: indicates the first phase of ventricular systole (Ciesla & Murdock 2000).
- *Peak systolic pressure*: this reflects maximum left ventricular systolic pressure.
- *Dicrotic notch*: reflects aortic valve closure (Garretson 2005). It is notably elevated in patients with increased peripheral resistance and decreased cardiac output.
- *Diastolic pressure*: reflects the degree of vasoconstriction or dilation in the arterial system.

Complications of arterial line insertion

Nurses need to be constantly alert to the possible complications of arterial line insertion. These include exsanguination, ischaemia distal to the cannula and tissue necrosis, inadvertent administration of drugs into the artery, air embolus and thrombosis (Table 5.5).

Monitoring priorities of a patient with an arterial line

The following measures should always be observed when a patient with an arterial line is being monitored:

- Ensure the tubing and cannula are secured.
- Clearly label the tubing 'arterial' to help prevent accidental arterial injection of drugs (Mallett & Dougherty 2000).
- Use a transparent dressing so that any dislodgement or disconnection will be immediately recognised.

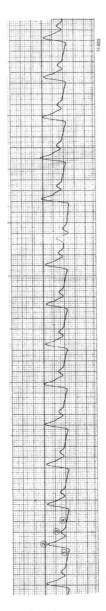

Fig. 5.3 Arterial waveform. 1. anacrotic notch; 2. peak systolic pressure; 3. dicrotic notch; 4. diastolic pressure.

Table 5.5 Summary of potential problems associated with an arterial cannula.

Problem	Cause	Action
'Dampened' trace (Fig. 5.4) leading to underestimated BP (blunt pressure peak, loss of dicrotic notch)	Loss of pressure or no fluid in the infusion pressure bag	Inflate pressure bag to 300 mmHg Check there is sufficient flushing fluid
	Thrombus/fibrin formation at tip of catheter	Withdraw blood and then flush catheter
	Air in tubing or transducer	Disconnect tubing from catheter and flush through to expel air before reconnecting If necessary, change transducer
	Too many three-way taps in the circuit	Remove excess taps
	Long length of tubing between catheter and transducer	Shorten tubing
	Poor position of limb, tip of catheter against vessel wall, kinked tubing	Manipulate catheter and/or limb to achieve a better trace
No arterial waveform (straight line)	Taps turned off to patient or transducer	Check taps are on to patient and transducer
	Disconnection of catheter	Check catheter site – reconnect immediately
	Disconnection of transducer cable to monitor	Check connections – reconnect
	Poor catheter position (tip against vessel wall) Asystole	Manipulate position, flush catheter Institute CPR
Backflow of blood from catheter towards transducer	Loose tap connection within the circuit	Check all connections are secure
	Flush bag pressure too low (below patient's BP)	Inflate bag to 300 mmHg pressure

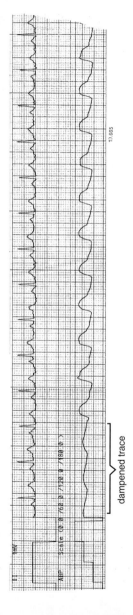

Fig. 5.4 Dampened arterial trace.

- Ensure that the limb is visible at all times to monitor perfusion and maintain a closed circuit.
- Regularly assess tissue perfusion distal to the cannula site. Thrombosis or the development of an adjacent haematoma could jeopardise arterial blood flow. If signs of poor tissue perfusion are present, e.g. if the limb becomes white, cold or painful, inform medical staff immediately – the line will need to be removed.
- Regularly assess the site for signs of infection. Replace dressing if soiled.
- Maintain a bag of 0.9% normal saline at a pressure of 300 mgHg to help maintain patency and change it following locally agreed protocols.
- Ensure all connections are secure. Exsanguination through an 18 FG cannula can lead to blood loss of 500 ml per minute (Gomersall & Oh 1997). Extra vigilance is required if the femoral artery has been used because the site will be covered up. If the cannula is transduced alarms should be appropriately set to alert the nurse to any disruption in the pressures indicating disconnection.
- Only competent practitioners should undertake arterial blood sampling.
- Use minimum amount of 'taps' to reduce the risk of infection, leakage and inadvertent drug administration.

Troubleshooting – flat arterial trace

If a flat arterial trace is observed on the monitor check the:

- patient is not in asystole
- circuit connections
- circuit for air bubbles and safely remove if present
- tubing in the circuit is not kinked
- flush bag has adequate fluid and a sufficient pressure is being maintained
- proximal joint as the cannula may be kinked or compressed against the vessel wall – repositioning the joint may be necessary
- patency of the arterial cannula by withdrawing blood
- patient's blood pressure manually

Once the problem has been rectified flush and re-zero line

Pulse contour analysis
Devices are now available which analyse the shape of the arterial waveform (pulse contour analysis): they can derive stroke volume and determine cardiac output (Gwinnutt 2006). The stroke volume is derived from the analysis of the systolic area of the arterial waveform, with corrections for the patient's age and heart rate (British Hypertension Society 2006). Calibration against a simultaneous method, e.g. thermodilution, enables pulse contour analysis to be used on peripheral arterial waveforms (British Hypertension Society 2006).

PRINCIPLES OF CENTRAL VENOUS PRESSURE MONITORING

Central venous pressure (CVP) reflects right atrial filling pressure or right ventricular preload (Druding 2000) and is dependent upon blood volume, vascular tone and cardiac function (Woodrow 2002). The normal CVP is 0–8 mmHg (Woodrow 2000). A low CVP reading usually indicates hypovolaemia while a high CVP reading has a number of causes, including hypervolaemia, cardiac failure and pulmonary embolism.

Indications for central venous catheters

Indications for central venous catheters include:

- fluid resuscitation
- drug and fluid administration
- parenteral feeding
- measurement of central venous pressure
- poor venous access
- cardiac pacing

(Woodrow 2002)

In the UK, approximately 200 000 central venous catheters are inserted each year (NICE 2002). The usual sites for insertion of central venous catheters are internal jugular (right and left) and subclavian (right or left). The latter is often the preferred site. Although the subclavian has more recognisable landmarks to aid the clinician there are fewer risks associated with the internal jugular. The femoral vein is sometimes used but generally only as a last resort because of the increased risk of infection (Woodrow 2002).

Central venous catheters can be single, triple, quadruple or quintuple lumened. Strict asepsis must be adhered to on insertion and following management as microorganisms that colonise catheter hubs and the skin adjacent to the insertion site are the source of most catheter-related bloodstream infections (Department of Health 2001).

There is recent evidence to suggest that antimicrobial-impregnated central venous catheters used short-term (<7 days) reduce the risk of catheter-related bloodstream infections (Mermel 2000), although these have only been recently available in the UK.

Central venous pressure (CVP) monitoring can be helpful in the assessment of cardiac function, circulating blood volume, vascular tone and the patient's response to treatment. However CVP can be influenced by a number of factors and should therefore be interpreted in combination with other systemic measurements. An isolated CVP measurement can be misleading; a trend in readings will demonstrate response to treatment and/or disease progression (Woodrow 2002) and is therefore of more value.

To help ensure validity of the measurements and accuracy of their interpretation, the patient's position should be constant (supine if possible) and the same point of reference (mid-axilla) should be used for each reading.

Methods of CVP monitoring

There are two methods of CVP monitoring:

- *manometer system*: enables intermittent readings and is less accurate than the transducer system and less frequently used
- *transducer system*: enables continuous readings which are displayed on a monitor (Gwinnutt 2006)

Procedure for CVP measurement using a manometer

1. Explain the procedure to the patient.
2. Ensure patency of the central venous catheter prior to the procedure – this can normally be ascertained by checking that the flush is working or by drawing blood back.

3. Position the patient supine, if possible. The same position should be used for each measurement to help ensure the trend of readings is accurate.
4. Align the manometer arm with the mid-axilla, ensuring that the 'bubble' is in between the lines on the spirit level. The reading on the manometer scale at this level should be zero (the baseline of the manometer scale is now level with the right atrium). Use the same point of reference for each measurement.
5. Turn the three-way tap off to the patient and on to the manometer. Check the fluid source, ensuring it is the correct solution to use (usually normal saline) and does not contain drugs.
6. Switch on the fluid source and slowly fill up the manometer tubing to above the expected reading. Care should be taken to ensure the manometer tubing fills up slowly. This will help avoid air bubbles which can lead to an inaccurate reading and prevent over-filling of, and spillage from, the manometer which is an infection risk (Mallett & Dougherty 2000).
7. Turn the three-way tap 'off' to the fluid source and 'on' to the patient. The fluid level in the manometer tubing should fall rapidly. This will allow fluid from the manometer to enter the right atrium.
8. Once the fluid level stops falling (it should be oscillating with the patient's respirations) the reading can then be taken using the lower reading.
9. Turn the three-way tap off to the patient (reconnect infusion fluids if appropriate).
10. Document the reading and report any changes or abnormalities.

Procedure for CVP measurement using a transducer

1. Explain the procedure to the patient.
2. Ensure patency of the central venous catheter prior to the procedure.
3. Position the patient, supine if possible. The same position should be used for each measurement.
4. Calibrate (zero) the monitor following the manufacturer's recommendations – this usually involves opening the system to

the atmosphere (off to the patient, open to air) and pressing a 'zero' button on the monitor; once zero is displayed the monitor has been calibrated). Zeroing a CVP ensures that the atmospheric pressure at the point of measurement is zero (Woodrow 2002).

5. Observe the CVP trace on the monitor. The waveform on the monitor should be slightly undulating in nature (Fig. 5.5), reflecting changes in right atrial pressure during the cardiac cycle.

6. Document the reading and report any changes and abnormalities (also calculate mean pressure reading).

The CVP waveform

The CVP waveform reflects changes in right atrial pressure during the cardiac cycle. Figure 5.5 depicts a typical CVP waveform and its configuration can be described as follows:

- *A wave: right atrial contraction (P wave on the ECG).* If the A wave is elevated the patient may have right ventricular failure or tricuspid stenosis.
- *C wave: tricuspid valve closure (follows QRS complex on the ECG).* The distance from A–C should correlate with the PR interval on the ECG.
- *V wave: pressure generated to the right atrium during ventricular contraction, despite the tricuspid valve being closed (latter part of the T wave on the ECG).* If the V wave is elevated the patient may have tricuspid valve disease.

Normal CVP measurements

Central venous pressure monitoring should normally show measurements as follows:

- 5–10 mmHg mid-axilla
- 7–14 cmH$_2$0 mid-axilla

(Woodrow 2002)

Troubleshooting

Hinds and Watson (1996) identified the following pitfalls with CVP monitoring:

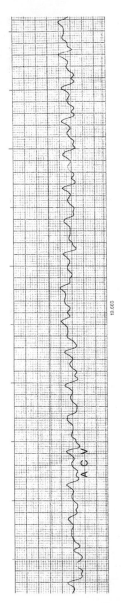

Fig. 5.5 CVP trace. A, C and V waves.

- *Occluded catheter*: this will result in a persistent high reading with a dampened trace. Ensure that the catheter is patent.
- *Incorrect calibration*: if a transducer and oscilloscope are used, the system should be calibrated following the manufacturer's recommendations.
- *Inconsistent procedure for measurements*: ensure consistent procedure (identical patient position and point of reference) for serial CVP measurements.
- *Infusion(s) in progress*: a falsely high CVP measurement will result if infusion(s) continue to be administered through the CVP catheter during the procedure. In addition if the infusion fluid contains vasoactive drugs, the resultant 'flush' can cause a sudden period of cardiac instability. Infusion(s) should be temporarily switched off while CVP measurement is undertaken (ideally all infusions should be administered through other lumens).
- *Catheter tip in the right ventricle*: this will result in an unexpected high pressure reading. If the patient is transduced the presenting waveform will confirm suspicions.
- *Respiratory oscillations*: measurements should be taken at end-expiration, especially if the patient is in respiratory distress or is being ventilated, as the CVP will be artificially higher because of positive intrathoracic pressure.

Complications following CVP line insertion

Nurses should be alert to the possibility of complications following central venous catheter insertion:

- malposition of the catheter (Czepizak *et al*. 1995) (Fig. 5.6)
- arterial puncture (Robinson *et al*. 1995)
- pneumothorax (Woodrow 2002)
- haemorrhage
- infection
- air emboli: although <20 ml of air rarely causes problems (Hudak *et al*. 1998) larger volumes of air could cause a pulmonary embolism and cardiac arrest
- thrombosis
- ventricular perforation
- cardiac arrhythmias

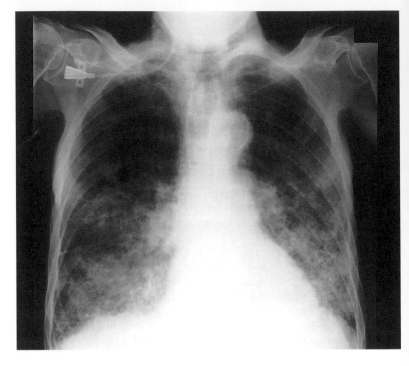

Fig. 5.6 Malposition of the CVP catheter – patient with known COPD and basal pulmonary fibrosis. The right subclavian line tip is pointing cranially with the tip in the internal jugular vein. (We are grateful to Louise Holland, Consultant Radiologist at the Manor Hospital Walsall for her assistance.)

Management of a patient with a central venous catheter

The precautions listed below should always be observed.

- Monitor the patient for signs of complications.
- Label central venous catheter with drugs/fluids, etc. being infused in order to minimise the risk of accidental bolus injection.
- If not in use, flush the cannula regularly to help prevent thrombosis. A 500 ml bag of 0.9% normal saline should be maintained

at a pressure of 300 mmHg and changed in accordance with locally agreed protocols.

- Ensure all connections are secure to prevent exsanguination, introduction of infection and air emboli.
- Observe the insertion site frequently for signs of infection. Transparent dressings should be used to permit continuous monitoring of the site. The incidence of central venous catheter related infection ranges from 4–18%. If infection of the central venous catheter is suspected blood cultures should be taken following removal of the line. The catheter tip should be sent for culture. The length of the indwelling catheter should be recorded and regularly monitored. The dressing should be changed as required, ensuring strict aseptic technique.
- Although the routine replacement of CVP lines is widespread in the UK (Cyna *et al.* 1998), this is not recommended as such practice is associated with a higher incidence of morbidity and mortality in critically ill patients. In addition replacing a CVP line is not only expensive and traumatic for the patient, but there is also an added risk of introducing an infection (Clemence *et al.* 1995). Central venous catheters should therefore only be removed when clinically indicated (O'Leary & Bihari 1998).
- Be alert to possible complications identified above.

PRINCIPLES OF PULMONARY ARTERY PRESSURE MONITORING

Pulmonary artery catheter

Since it was first described by Swan and Ganz in the 1970s, the pulmonary artery (PA) catheter, which is also known as a multi-lumen directional flow catheter (Fig. 5.7), has been widely used for the diagnosis and treatment of critically ill patients.

It can be used to evaluate cardiac function and to detect problems in the pulmonary vasculature and enables the clinician to optimise cardiac output and delivery of oxygen whilst minimising the risk of pulmonary oedema; it also allows the rational use of vasoactive and inotropic drugs (Hinds & Watson 1999). The use of the PA catheter is not without risk. Although it has been common in the ICU environment in the last 30 years there have

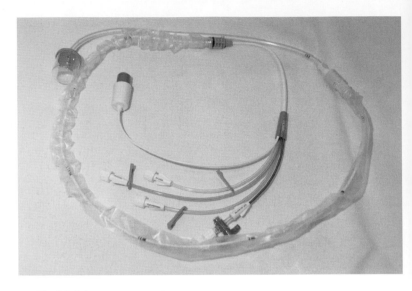

Fig. 5.7 Pulmonary artery catheter.

been doubts about its safety. However, a large multi-centre randomised controlled trial (Harvey *et al*. 2005) concluded that there was no clear evidence of benefit or harm to the critically ill patient managed with a PA catheter. The use of PA catheters should be limited to experienced, well trained clinicians familiar with the interpretation of data derived from the catheter, who are able to adjust treatment based on the results obtained.

Because of doubts surrounding the efficacy of PA catheters, less invasive methods of measuring cardiac output have been developed and these will be discussed later.

Indications

Use of PA pressure measurement is indicated for:

- assessment of circulatory volume and fluid management in impaired right or left ventricular function or pulmonary hypertension

- cardiac output measurements
- mixed venous saturation measurements
- diagnosis of ventricular septal defect
- post cardiac surgery

(Gomersall & Oh 1997)

Waveform as pulmonary artery catheter passes from the vena cava to the pulmonary artery

Figure 5.8 depicts the pressure traces seen as a pulmonary artery catheter passes from the vena cava to the pulmonary artery. Pulmonary vasculature is more compliant than the systemic vessels, consequently pulmonary pressures are lower (Table 5.5) (Woodrow 2000). Pulmonary hypertension is common in ICU patients, e.g. those with acute respiratory distress syndrome (ARDS). If the pulmonary artery pressure is low despite a high CVP this is indicative of right-sided heart failure (Woodrow 2000).

Pressures

Using a pulmonary catheter it is possible to measure the pressures in the right atrium (RA), right ventricle (RV) and pulmonary artery (PA) (Table 5.5):

- RA pressure: during ventricular filling is 0–8 mmHg
- RV pressure: end diastolic pressure is 0–8 mmHg, systolic pressure 15–30 mmHg
- PA pressure: diastolic 5–15 mmHg, systolic 15–30 mmHg

A high diastolic pressure indicates right heart failure, pulmonary hypertension or tamponade. High PA pressure indicates left ventricular failure (LVF) or pulmonary hypertension, low PA pressure is suggestive of hypovolaemia.

Cardiac index (CI) is cardiac output indexed to individual body surface area. Normal is between 2.4 and 4 l/min/m^2 (Druding 2000). These readings may never be completely precise as it is very difficult to weigh and measure a very sick patient accurately. The relevance, however, is in the trend of results that the PA catheter facilitates and the response to treatment administered.

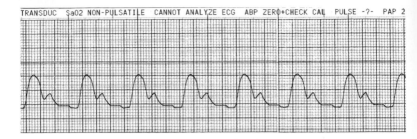

Fig. 5.8 Pressure traces seen as the pulmonary artery catheter passes from the vena cava to the pulmonary artery.

Pulmonary artery wedge pressure (PAWP)

If the balloon is inflated in the branch of the pulmonary artery, the pressure at the tip of the catheter will reflect the pressure distal to it, i.e. left atrial and ventricular pressure which is in direct correlation to left-sided heart preload (Druding 2000).

Procedure

1. Explain the procedure to the patient.
2. Watching the monitor at the same time, slowly inflate the balloon until the characteristic flattened waveform is identified (Fig. 5.8). The balloon is now 'wedged', i.e. it is occluding the blood flow in a branch of the pulmonary artery.
3. Stop inflating the balloon and allow the trace to run for three respiratory cycles (very important).
4. Freeze the monitor screen and deflate the balloon rapidly.
5. Ascertain the wedge pressure by aligning the cursor control on the monitor to the correct position on the waveform (end expiration).
6. Unfreeze the monitor screen and ensure the pulmonary artery waveform is present.

Precautions

Care should be taken to observe the following precautions:

- Do not leave the balloon inflated for longer than three respiratory cycles (15 seconds).

- Do not inflate more than 1.5 ml of air into the balloon.
- Do not flush the catheter if the balloon is inflated.
- If the trace rises sharply during balloon inflation, then the catheter is over-wedged.

Limitations
PAWP does not accurately reflect left atrial and ventricular pressure in:

- pulmonary venous obstruction
- mitral stenosis
- left atrial myxoma (very rare)

Normal wedge range is 5–15 mmHg (Woodrow 2000) and should correlate with the pulmonary artery diastolic pressure; a high reading may signify LVF, mitral insufficiency or fluid overload, whereas a low reading may signify hypovolaemia.

SVR is the measurement of afterload and a critical measurement in the diagnosis and treatment of sepsis. Normal SVR is 900–1400 dynes.s/cm^{-5}. Systemic vascular resistance index (SVRI) is indexed to body surface area calculated from weight and height.

Complications
Complications resulting following PA catheter use include:

- cardiac arrhythmias
- thrombosis
- pulmonary infarction
- rupture of the pulmonary artery – often associated with balloon inflation during measuring the wedge pressure (Leeper 1995)
- myocardial perforation (Daily & Schroeder 1989)
- knotting of the catheter (Tan *et al.* 1997)

CARDIAC OUTPUT STUDIES

Thermodilution
Thermodilution is a method for measuring cardiac output. To assess progress towards desired treatment goals it is important

that readings are taken following interventions, e.g. titration of vasoactive or inotropic drugs or fluid bolus. This process involves a rapid injection of a measured amount of cold fluid (usually 5–10 ml of 5% dextrose) into the right atrium through the proximal lumen of the PA catheter. Its dilution by the blood is calculated by serial changes in PA temperature as the fluid bolus travels through the heart. The cardiac output is calculated on the basis of the temperature change: the rise in solution temperature is inversely related to the functioning of the heart.

Indications
Thermodilution is indicated in clinical situations where the assessment of volaemic status and cardiac output along with haemodynamic variables will help in the diagnosis and management. For example:

- management and diagnosis of all forms of shock
- impaired right or left ventricular function as seen in cardiac failure
- measurement of cardiac output
- measurement of mixed venous saturation
- diagnosis of ventricular septal defect

Procedure

1. Explain the procedure to the patient.
2. Draw up the injection fluid.
3. Ensure that the temperature of injection fluid is lower than body temperature.
4. Flush the proximal port with the injection fluid; the injection fluid displayed on the monitor should be within the accepted range for the monitoring system.
5. Ensure that the monitor is ready.
6. Press the start button on the monitor and inject 5–10 ml smoothly within 4 seconds (do not hold the syringe barrel, as this could warm the injection fluid). Approximately 15 seconds later, the cardiac output measurement will be displayed on the monitor. After about 45 seconds, the monitor will display 'ready' again.

7. Press the start button again and repeat the above procedure. At least three measurements should be made and an average of the three readings calculated.

Troubleshooting

The following problems are associated with thermodilution cardiac output measurements (Adam & Osborne 1997):

- *Difficulty injecting the solution*: the tube may be kinked or occluded or the catheter tip may be positioned against the vessel wall. Unkink, reposition or replace catheter as necessary.
- *Blood temperature not displayed*: the thermistor may be faulty or may have a fibrin growth attached. Replace the catheter if necessary.
- *Injection fluid temperature not displayed*: replace the faulty temperature probe.
- *Major discrepancies in serial measurements*: possible causes include poor injection technique, cardiac arrhythmias (causing varying stroke volumes), and vascular disease causing turbulent blood and patient movement. Adhere to procedure described above, do not inject during arrhythmic episodes and limit patient movement during injection.
- *Inappropriately high cardiac output measurements*: possible causes include incorrect injection fluid volume (usually too little or leaking connection), injection fluid temperature too low, poor injection technique and computer error. Adhere to the procedure described above and if indicated check the computer.
- *Inappropriately low cardiac output measurements*: possible causes include incorrect injection fluid volume (usually too much), injection fluid temperature too high, start button on the monitor pressed after starting the injection, computer error, prolonged injection time and concomitant fluid infusion through the distal lumen. Adhere to the procedure described above and if indicated check the computer.

Mixed venous oxygen saturation

Mixed venous oxygen saturation (SVO_2) represents the amount of oxygen which remains after perfusion of the capillary beds and is an indicator of the balance between oxygen delivery and oxygen consumption (Takala 1997). SVO_2 measurements, which can be used as a guide to tissue perfusion, are directly proportional to cardiac output, haemoglobin and oxygen saturation levels and inversely with the metabolic rate (Gomersall & Oh 1997).

- SVO_2 75%: normal.
- $SVO_2 \leq 75\%$: low. If the oxygen delivery drops or if tissue oxygen demand rises this can lead to a low measurement. If $SVO_2 < 30\%$ then oxygen delivery is insufficient to meet the oxygen needs of the tissues.
- $SVO_2 \geq 75\%$: high, can be difficult to interpret. Causes include sepsis, hypothermia, cyanide poisoning, left to right cardiac shunts (Gomersall & Oh 1997).

Methods for SVO₂ measurements
SVO_2 measurement may be performed in two ways:

- *intermittent* blood sampling from the distal PA catheter or *continuously* through a fibreoptic PA catheter
- a co-oximeter is also required because blood gas machines are unable to calculate lower SVO_2

Non-invasive methods of measuring cardiac output
Because of the invasive nature of PA catheters and their associated complications, it may be preferable to use non-invasive methods if available, to measure cardiac function.

NICO®
NICO® is a non-invasive device (Fig. 5.9) which calculates cardiac output by a modified Fick equation, based on partial carbon dioxide rebreathing. Cardiac output data are derived from sensors which measure flow, airway pressure and carbon dioxide concentration. Because of this use of the NICO is limited to the patient who is mechanically ventilated.

PiCCO®
PiCCO® is continuous pulse contour cardiac analysis and provides derived haemodynamic data via a femoral or axillary artery catheter and a central venous catheter.

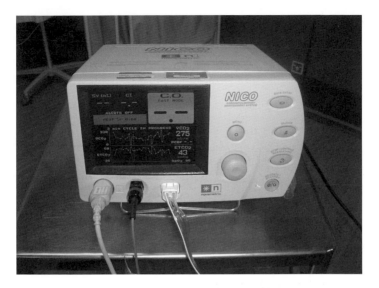

Fig. 5.9 Non-invasive cardiac output monitor.

Transoesophageal Doppler (TOE)

This involves introducing a Doppler into the oesophagus and echo imaging of blood flow turbulence through the aorta is demonstrated. It is accurate within 2.9% of thermodilution cardiac output studies and the majority of measurements are underestimates (Hinds & Watson 1999). It is only suitable for sedated patients and can cause oesophageal trauma (Valtier *et al*. 1998).

SCENARIOS

Scenario 1

Susan, a 45-year-old woman with known gallstones, was admitted to hospital with a history of right upper quadrant pain, pyrexia, vomiting and malaise. Her vital signs were:

Continued

BP 115/55 mmHg
HR 100/min
Respiratory rate 24/min
SpO_2 97% on air
Temperature 37.6°C

A provisional diagnosis of cholecystitis was made and she was commenced on an IV infusion to maintain hydration, an analgesic regime and cefotaxime 2 g IV TDS and metronidazole 500 mg IV TDS.

On day two of her admission Susan's condition deteriorated. She complained of feeling very unwell. On examination she was flushed, warm to the touch with warm peripheries. Her vital signs were:

BP 100/50 mmHg
HR 120/min
Respiratory rate 30/min
SpO_2 93% on air
Temperature 38.5°C

High-flow oxygen was commenced via a non-rebreathe mask and IV fluid increased to 150 ml/hr.

Susan continued to deteriorate and was transferred to the ICU for further management. On admission to ICU Susan was becoming confused and agitated. She was continually trying to remove her oxygen mask and desaturating as a result. The decision was made to electively sedate and ventilate her. On rapid sequence induction Susan developed severe hypotension which required fluid resuscitation and bolus doses of ephedrine. When she had stabilised intravenous access was established via a quadruple-lumen central venous catheter and an arterial line sited. Susan continued to demonstrate haemodynamic instability and was commenced on an infusion of nor-adrenaline via the central venous catheter. Because of her rapid deterioration and suspected septic shock a PA catheter was inserted and the following readings obtained:

Pulmonary capillary wedge pressure (PCWP) 10 mmHg
Cardiac output (CO) 3.0 l/min
Cardiac Index (CI) 2.1 l/min/m²
Stroke volume index (SVI) 45 ml/beat/m²
Systemic vascular resistance (SVR) 1200 dynes.sec/cm⁻⁵
CVP 3 mmHg

The PA catheter results confirmed a reduced cardiac output secondary to septic shock.

Scenario 2

Gordon, a 54-year-old man, presented with a short duration of severe central chest pain with associated nausea and diaphoresis. He was given aspirin 300 mg orally and sublingual glyceryl trinitrate (GTN) prior to arriving at the Emergency Department. In the Emergency Department he was commenced on oxygen and given IV morphine 2 mg. Blood was taken for cardiac biomarkers and urea and electrolytes. In the Emergency Department 12-lead ECG diagnosis confirmed a non ST segment acute coronary syndrome (NSTEAC). As this does not require reperfusion therapy Gordon was immediately transferred to the coronary care unit (CCU).

His observations were within normal limits, he was pain free, warm and well perfused. Shortly after admission he suddenly developed a broad complex tachycardia, rate 180/min. He was conscious, what would you do?

The patient is conscious therefore he must have a pulse (if he was pulseless, CPR and rapid defibrillation would be required). If not already, administer oxygen, secure IV access and establish whether the patient is haemodynamically compromised. Are there any adverse signs? (E.g. systolic blood pressure <90 mmHg, chest pain, heart failure, rapid rate >150/min (Resuscitation Council UK 2000)).

On examination Mr Smith's pulse is weak, rapid (180/min) and thready. His blood pressure has fallen to 70 mmHg systolic, he is cold, pale and clammy and his conscious level is deteriorating. What would you do?

He is severely haemodynamically compromised and requires urgent treatment, e.g. cardioversion. If the patient had not been compromised, drugs, e.g. amiodarone or lignocaine, would have probably been the first choice of treatment. Any electrolyte imbalance would also need to be treated.

CONCLUSION

Haemodynamic monitoring is central to the care of a critically ill patient. It helps to establish a precise diagnosis, determine appropriate therapy and monitor the response to that therapy. In particular the various methods of haemodynamic monitoring can assist in the early recognition and treatment of shock. Early recognition and prompt treatment of such disorders improves outcomes. It is always preferable to utilise the least invasive, yet most accurate technique available to reduce the risk of complications for the patient. Users of monitoring devices must be familiar with the operation of and how to trouble shoot, which will minimise the risk of erroneous results.

REFERENCES

Adam, S.K. & Osborne, S. (1997) *Critical Care Nursing: Science and Practice*. Oxford University Press, Oxford.

Bridges, E.J. & Dukes, M.S. (2005) Cardiovascular aspects of septic shock. Pathophysiology, monitoring and treatment. *Critical Care Nurse* **25** (2), 14–40.

British Hypertension Society (2006) *Blood pressure measurement*. www.bhsoc.org (accessed 16/09/06).

CEN European Committee for Standardisation (1995) *EN 1060-1 Non-invasive sphygmomanometers: general requirements*. British Standards Institution, London.

Ciesla, N.D. & Murdock, K. (2000) Lines, tubes, catheters and physiologic monitoring in the ICU. *Cardiopulmonary Physical Therapy Journal* **11** (1), 16–25.

Clemence, M., Walker, D. & Forr, B. (1995) Central venous catheter practices: results of a survey. *American Journal of Infection Control* **23** (1), 5–12.

Collins, T. (2000) Understanding Shock. *Nursing Standard* **14** (49), 35–40.

Cyna, A.M., Hovenden, J.L., Lehmann, A. *et al*. (1998) Routine replacement of central venous catheters: telephone survey of intensive care units in mainland Britain. *British Medical Journal* **316**, 1944–1945.

Czepizak, C.A., O'Callaghan, J.M. & Venus, B. (1995) Evaluation of formulas for optimal positioning of central venous catheters. *Chest* **107**, 1662–1664.

Daily, E.K. & Schroeder, J.S. (1989) *Techniques in Bedside Hemodynamic Monitoring* 4th edn. C.V. Mosby, London.

Department of Health (2001) Guidelines for preventing infections associated with the insertion and maintenance of central venous catheters. *Journal of Hospital Infection* **47** (supplement), S47–S67.

Diehl-Oplinger, L. & Kaminski, M.F. (2004) Choosing the right fluid to counter hypovolaemic shock. *Nursing* **34** (3), 52–54.

Druding, M.C. (2000) Integrating haemodynamic monitoring and physical assessment. *Dimensions of Critical Care Nursing* **19** (4), 25–30.

Duke, G.J., Briedis, J.H. & Weaver, R.A. (1994) Renal support in critically ill patients: low dose dopamine or low dose dobutamine? *Critical Care Medicine* **22**, 1919–1925.

European Society of Intensive Care Medicine Expert Panel (1991) The use of the pulmonary artery catheter. *Intensive Care Medicine* **17**, 1–8.

Garretson, S. (2005) Haemodynamic monitoring: arterial catheters. *Nursing Standard* **19** (31), 55–63.

Giuliano, K.K. (2006) Continuous physiologic monitoring and the identification of sepsis. *AACN Advanced Critical Care* **17** (2), 215–223.

Gomersall, C. & Oh, T. (1997) Haemodynamic monitoring. In: T. Oh, ed. *Intensive Care Manual* 4th edn. Butterworth Heinemann, Oxford.

Graham, C. & Parke, T. (2005) Critical care in the emergency department: shock and circulatory support. *Emergency Medicine Journal* **22**, 17–21.

Green, J.H. (1991) *An Introduction to Human Physiology*. Oxford Medical Publications, Oxford.

Gwinnutt, C. (2006) *Clinical Anaesthesia* 2nd edn. Blackwell Publishing, Oxford.

Hand, H. (2001) Shock. *Nursing Standard* **15** (48), 45–52.

Harvey, S., Harrison, D.A. & Singer, M. (2005) Assessment of the clinical effect of pulmonary artery catheters in the management of patients in intensive care (PAC-Man): a randomized controlled trial. *Lancet* **366**, 472–477.

Henderson, N. (1997) Central venous lines. *Nursing Standard* **11** (42), 49–56.

Hinds, C.J. & Watson, D. (1996) *Intensive Care, a concise textbook* 2nd edn. W.B. Saunders, London.

Hinds, C.J. & Watson, D. (1999) ABC of intensive care: circulatory support. *British Medical Journal* **318**, 1749–1752.

Hudak, C.M., Gallo, B.M. & Morton, P.G. (1998) *Critical Care Nursing: a holistic approach* 7th edn. Lippincott, New York.

Jones, C. (2006) Central venous catheter infection in adults in acute hospital settings. *British Journal of Nursing* **15** (7), 362–368.

Leach, R. (2004) Critical Care Medicine at a Glance. Blackwell Publishing, Oxford.

Lee, R. & Branch, J. (1997) Postoperative cardiac intensive care. In: T. Oh, ed. *Intensive Care Manual* 4th edn. Butterworth-Heinemann, Oxford.

Leeper, B. (1995) Ask the experts. *Critical Care Nurse* **15**, 82–83.

Mallett, J. & Dougherty, L. (2000) eds. *The Royal Marsden Hospital Manual of Clinical Nursing Procedures*. Blackwell Science, Oxford.

Mermel, L. (2000) Prevention of intravascular catheter-related infection. *Annals of Internal Medicine* **32** (5), 391–402.

Mosby Publishers (1998) *Mosby's Medical, Nursing and Allied Health Dictionary* 5th edn. Mosby, London.

Newell, R.W. (2005) Assessing, treating and managing patients with sepsis. *Nursing Standard* **19** (50), 56–64.

NICE (2002) *NICE guidance on the use of ultrasound locating devices for placing central venous catheters*. NICE, London.

O'Brien, E., Beevers, D. & Marshall, H. (1995) *ABC of Hypertension*. BMJ Books, London.

O'Leary, M. & Bihari, D. (1998) Central venous catheters – time for change? *British Medical Journal* **316**, 1918–1919.

Resuscitation Council UK (2000) *Advanced Life Support Manual* 4th edn. Resuscitation Council UK, London.

Robinson, J.F., Robinson, W.A., Cohn, H. *et al.* (1995) Perforation of the great vessels during central venous line placement. *Archives of Internal Medicine* **155**, 1225–1228.

Robson, W. & Newell, J. (2005) Assessing, treating and managing patients with sepsis. *Nursing Standard* **19** (50), 56–64.

Skowronski, G. (1997) Circulator shock. In: T. Oh, ed. *Intensive Care Manual* 4th edn. Butterworth-Heinemann, Oxford.

Smith, G. (2000) Devices for blood pressure measurement. *Professional Nurse* **15** (5), 337–340.

Starling, E.H. (1918) *The Law of the Heart*. Linacre Lecture, London.

Swan, H.J.C. & Ganz, W. (1974) Guidelines for use of balloon-tipped catheters. *American Journal of Cardiology* **34**, 119–120.

Takala, J. (1997) Monitoring oxygenation. In: T. Oh, ed. *Intensive Care Manual*, 4th edn. Butterworth Heinemann, Oxford.

Tan, C. *et al.* (1997) A technique to remove knotted pulmonary artery catheters. *Anaesthesia and Intensive Care* **25** (2), 160–162.

Torrance, C. & Semple, M. (1997) Blood pressure measurement. *Nursing Times* **93** (38), suppl. 1–2.

Valtier, B., Cholley, B., Belot, J.-P. *et al.* (1998) Non-invasive monitoring of cardiac output in critically ill patients using transoesophageal doppler. *American Journal of Respiratory and Critical Care Medicine* **158** (1), 77–83.

Woodrow, P. (2000) *Intensive Care Nursing, A Framework for Practice*. Routledge, London.

Woodrow, P. (2002) Central venous catheters and central venous pressure. *Nursing Standard* **16** (26), 45–51.

Monitoring Neurological Function

6

INTRODUCTION

Altered level of consciousness is common in the critically ill patient (Smith 2003). Changes in neurological function can be rapid and dramatic, or subtle developing over a period of minutes, hours, days or even longer (Aucken & Crawford 1998). In patients with a head injury or other cerebral insult, monitoring neurological function is essential in order to recognise and treat complications promptly and improve prognosis (Hinds & Watson 1996). It can also provide an indication to the function of other systems, e.g. in renal failure confusion could be a sign of rising blood urea levels.

Monitoring neurological function requires accurate assessment and correct interpretation of observed data (Bassett & Makin 2000). It is important to take into account the effects of any administered medications, e.g. sedatives and paralysing agents (Woodrow 2000a), alcohol consumption, the patient's clinical condition and whether there is a history of head injury.

The aim of this chapter is to understand the principles of monitoring neurological function.

LEARNING OBJECTIVES

At the end of the chapter the reader will be able to:

❏ define *consciousness*
❏ describe the *AVPU* assessment of consciousness
❏ discuss the use of the *Glasgow Coma Scale*
❏ describe *pupillary assessment*
❏ discuss the principles of *intracranial pressure monitoring*

❏ discuss the principles of *jugular venous bulb oxygen saturation monitoring*
❏ outline the monitoring of *sedation*
❏ outline the monitoring of *pain* and *pain relief*

DEFINITION OF CONSCIOUSNESS

The patient's level of consciousness has been described as the degree of their arousal and awareness (Geraghty 2005). It is dependent upon the interaction of the ascending reticular activating system situated in the brainstem and the cerebral hemispheres. Any disruption in this communication process will result in impaired consciousness (Bassett & Makin 2000).

The manifestation of impaired or absent consciousness implies an underlying brain dysfunction (Geraghty 2005). Various scales have been designed to describe levels of consciousness (Geraghty 2005) however, the National Institute for Clinical Excellence (NICE 2003) recommends the Glasgow Coma Scale (GCS) be used to assess all patients with head injuries. Definitions of impaired consciousness are listed in Table 6.1. It is not possible to measure consciousness directly. It can only be assessed by observing the patient's behavioural response to different stimuli (Waterhouse 2005).

AVPU ASSESSMENT

The most important aspect of any neurological assessment is the level of consciousness because this is the most sensitive indicator of neurological deterioration (Waterhouse 2005). A rapid neurological assessment can be carried out using the AVPU method (Resuscitation Council UK 2006). AVPU is a mnemonic for a simple, rapid and effective neurological scoring system which quantifies the response to stimulation and assesses the level of consciousness. It is ideal in the emergency situation when a rapid assessment of conscious level is required. AVPU stands for:

Alert
Responsive to **v**erbal stimulation
Responsive to **p**ainful stimulation
Unresponsive.

Table 6.1 Definitions of impaired consciousness.

Condition	Definition
Consciousness	Awareness of self and environment
Confusion	Reduced awareness, disorientation
Delirium	Disorientation, fear, irritability, misperception, hallucination
Obtundation	Reduced alertness, psychomotor retardation, drowsiness
Stupor	Unresponsiveness with arousal only by vigorous and repeated stimuli
Coma	Unarousable unresponsiveness
Vegetative state	Prolonged coma (>1 month), some preservation of brainstem and motor reflexes
Akinetic mutism	Prolonged coma with apparent alertness and flaccid motor tone
Locked-in state	Total paralysis below third cranial nerve nuclei; normal or impaired mental function

Reprinted from *Intensive Care Manual*, T. Oh, 4th edn, © 1997, with permission from Elsevier Inc.

ACDU ASSESSMENT

ACDU is an acronym to describe another assessment system which may be useful as a component of early warning scoring sytems (McNarry & Goldhill 2004):

Alert
Confused
Drowsy
Unresponsive.

THE GLASGOW COMA SCALE

The Glasgow Coma Scale (GCS) was originally developed to grade the severity and outcome of traumatic head injury (Teasdale & Jennett 1974). It is now used worldwide to assess the level of consciousness (Mallett & Dougherty 2000) and allows:

- *standardisation* of the clinical observations of patients with impaired consciousness

- *progress monitoring* of patients undergoing intracranial surgery with minimal variation and subjectivity in the clinical assessment
- an *indication* to prognosis

(Shah 1999)

The Glasgow Coma Scale assesses the two aspects of consciousness:

- *arousal* or *wakefulness*: being aware of the environment
- *awareness*: demonstrating an understanding of what the practitioner has said through an ability to perform tasks

The 15-point scale assesses the patient's level of consciousness by evaluating three behavioural responses: eye opening, verbal response and motor response (Fairley 2005; Waterhouse 2005). Within each category, each level of response is allocated a numerical value, on a scale of increasing neurological deterioration (Waterhouse 2005). By assigning a numerical value to the level of response to the individual criteria in each section, three figures are obtained which add up to a maximum score of 15 and a minimum of three. Coma is said to exist when GCS is <8 (Albarran & Price 1998). A total score of 12 or less should give rise for concern (Woodrow 2000b). A reduction in motor score by one or an overall deterioration of two, is significant and should be reported (Cree 2003; NICE 2003). Although aggregate scores are often documented, the weighting of scores between eye, verbal and motor responses remains untested (Woodrow 2000b). Therefore documenting responses individually may provide a clearer indication of remaining functions and deficits (Waterhouse 2005). The neurological observation chart depicted in Fig. 6.1 incorporates the GCS.

The GCS is simple to use, requires no special equipment and is a good predictor of outcome (Woodrow 2000a). It can be used by different observers and still produce a consistent assessment and has been found to be reliable and easy to use (Cree 2003). However, as with other scoring systems, the GCS is liable to subjectivity (Woodrow 2000a) and should only be used as an aid to patient assessment (Adam & Osborne 1999). Intra-observer differences in measuring the GCS may occur unless training in

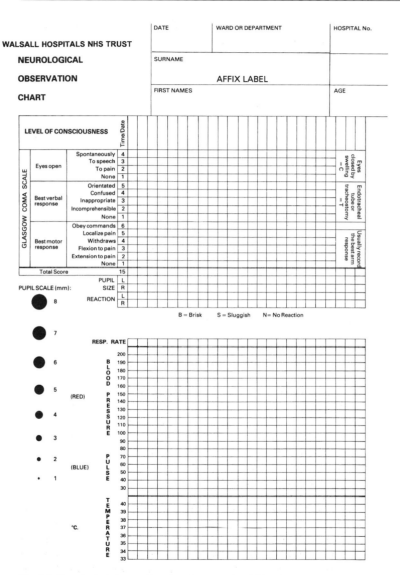

Fig. 6.1 Neurological observation chart incorporating GCS (Walsall Hospitals NHS Trust).

153

the use of the tool has been given to prevent inaccurate and inconsistent recordings which could have a detrimental effect on the patient (Mooney & Comerford 2003). It has therefore been suggested that at shift handover assessment of the patient's GCS by nurses on both shifts should be undertaken in order to identify any discrepancies (Woodrow 2000b).

The frequency of GCS monitoring should be individualised to the patient's needs (Woodrow 2000b). Instead of stressing the numerical score attached to each response, it is far better to define the responses in descriptive terms.

There are difficulties with using the GCS on an ICU (Price 1996), particularly in sedated, ventilated head-injured patients. The GCS is not designed to assess sedation scores but how well the brain is functioning (Cree 2003). Differences in scores of two or more have been reported on the same patients by different practitioners (Holdgate 2006) which reiterates the recommendation that clinical decisions should not solely be based upon GCS (Holdgate 2006) but that GCS be used as a component of monitoring neurological function.

Behavioural responses assessed

The three behavioural responses assessed are:

- eye opening
- verbal response
- motor response

Each will now be discussed in turn.

Eye opening

Assessment of eye opening involves the evaluation of arousal, the first aspect of consciousness. If the patient's eyes are closed, their state of arousal is assessed according to the degree of stimulation required to secure eye opening. Eye opening (arousal) is always the first measurement undertaken as part of the GCS because without it cognition cannot occur (Aucken & Crawford 1998). If the patient's eyes are swollen, opening them may not be possible (Mallett & Dougherty 2000). The scoring is as follows:

- Score 4 = spontaneously: eyes open without the need for speech or touch (Fairley 2005); optimum response.

- Score 3 = to speech: eyes open in response to a verbal stimulus (usually the patient's name) without touching the patient (Waterhouse 2005). Begin at normal volume and raise your voice if necessary using clear commands (Fairley 2005).
- Score 2 = to pain: eyes open in response to central pain only, e.g. trapezium squeeze, suborbital pressure (recommended), sternal rub (Table 6.2). N.B. Painful stimuli should only be employed if the patient fails to respond to firm and clear commands (Mallett & Dougherty 2000).
- Score 1 = no response: no eye opening despite verbal and central pain stimulus.

*N.B. Record 'C' if the patient is unable to open the eyes due to swelling, ptosis or a dressing.

Verbal response

Assessment of verbal response involves the evaluation of awareness, the second aspect of consciousness. Comprehension of what the practitioner has said and functioning areas of the higher centres and ability to articulate and express a reply are being evaluated (Waterhouse 2005). Dysphasia or inability to speak can be caused by any damage to the speech centres in the brain, e.g. following intracranial surgery or head injury.

It is important to ascertain the patient's acuity of hearing and understanding of language prior to assessing this response (Adam

Table 6.2 Central painful stimuli.

Stimulus	Technique
Trapezium squeeze	Using the thumb and index finger pinch approximately 5 cm of the trapezius muscle (between the head and shoulders) and twist (Woodward 1997)
Suborbital pressure	Running a finger along the supraorbital margin (boney ridge along the top of the eye) it is possible to identify a notch or groove – applying pressure here causes a headache-type pain. Sometimes it may cause the patient to grimace, leading to closing rather than opening of the eyes. N.B. should not be used if the patient has facial fractures
Sternal rub	Grinding the sternum with the knuckles. N.B. alternate with other methods because of marking the skin.

& Osborne 1999). The lack of speech may not always indicate a falling level of consciousness (Mallett & Dougherty 2000). In addition some patients may require a lot of stimulation to maintain their concentration while answering questions. The amount of stimulation required should be documented as part of baseline assessment (Aucken & Crawford 1998). The scoring is as follows:

- Score 5 = orientated: the patient can tell the practitioner who they are, where they are and the day, the current year and month (avoid using the day of the week or date).
- Score 4 = confused: the patient can hold a conversation with the practitioner, but cannot answer the preceding questions accurately (Fairley 2005).
- Score 3 = inappropriate words: the patient tends to use single words more than sentences and conversational exchange is absent (Fairley 2005).
- Score 2 = incomprehensible sounds: the patient's response is made up of incomprehensible sounds such as moans or groans (Mooney & Comerford 2003) but no discernable words. A verbal stimulus together with a pain stimulus may be needed to get a response from the patient. This type of patient is not aware of their surroundings (Mooney & Comerford 2003).
- Score 1 = no response: no response from the patient despite both verbal or physical stimuli (Fairley 2005).

*N.B. Record 'D' if the patient is dysphasic and 'T' if the patient has a tracheal or tracheostomy tube in situ.

Motor response

The motor response is designed to ascertain the patient's ability to obey a command and to localise, withdraw or assume abnormal body positions in response to a painful stimulus (Adam & Osborne 1999). If the patient does not respond by obeying commands the response to a painful stimulus should then be assessed.

In the past the application of a peripheral painful stimulus (pressure applied to fingernail bed) has been advocated (Teasdale & Jennett 1974). However this can be traumatic and is no longer recommended. In addition a peripheral stimulus may only elicit a spinal reflex which does not involve cerebral function (Shah 1999). It can cause patients to pull their fingers away from the source of pain; only a central painful stimulus will demonstrate localisation to pain (Waterhouse 2005).

A true localising response involves the patient bringing an arm up to chin level, to pull an oxygen mask off for instance (Waterhouse 2005). To elicit this response the trapezium squeeze, supraorbital ridge pressure or pressure on the jaw margin are recommended. To avoid soft tissue injury the stimulus should be applied for no more than 10 seconds and released (Waterhouse 2005). In addition, when applying a stimulus, it is best practice to start off with light pressure and increase to elicit a response (Sheppard & Wright 2000).

- Score 6 = obeys commands: ask the patient to stick his tongue out; never ask a patient just to squeeze your hand as this could elicit a primitive grasp response, ensure you ask them to let go. As it is important to establish that the response is not just a reflex movement, it is important to ask the patient to carry out two different commands (Bassett & Makin 2000).
- Score 5 = localises to central pain, if the patient does not respond to verbal stimuli: the patient purposely moves an arm in an attempt to remove the cause of the pain. Supraorbital ridge pressure is considered to be the most reliable technique as this is less likely to be misinterpreted (Fairley 2005).
- Score 4 = withdrawing from pain: the patient flexes or bends arm towards the source of the pain but fails to locate the source of the pain (Waterhouse 2005). There is no wrist rotation.
- Score 3 = flexion to pain: the patient flexes or bends the arm. It is characterised by internal rotation and adduction of the shoulder and flexion of the elbow and is much slower than normal flexion (Fairley 2005).
- Score 2 = extension to pain: the patient extends the arm by straightening the elbow, sometimes associated with internal shoulder and wrist rotation, sometimes referred to as decerebrate posture (Waterhouse 2005).
- Score 1 = no response: no response to central painful stimuli.

Best practice – application of painful stimuli

Painful stimuli should only be employed if the patient fails to respond to firm and clear commands

To evaluate cerebral function, apply a central not peripheral stimulus, e.g. trapezium squeeze, supraorbital ridge pressure or pressure on the jaw margin

When applying a stimulus, start off with light pressure and increase to elicit a response

To avoid soft tissue injury no stimulus should be applied for more than 10 seconds

---

PUPILLARY ASSESSMENT

Although pupillary assessment is not part of the GCS, it is an essential adjunct to it, especially when consciousness is impaired (Bersten *et al.* 2003). Pupillary reaction is an assessment of the third cranial nerve (oculomotor nerve) which controls constriction of the pupil. Compression of this nerve will result in fixed dilated pupils (Fairley 2005). GCS may be difficult to assess in sedated ventilated patients, and then the pupillary reaction test indicates much about the patient's neurological status (Cree 2003). Any changes in pupil reaction, size or shape, together with other neurological signs, are an indication of raised intracranial pressure (ICP) and compression of the optic nerve (Mooney & Comerford 2003).

Prior to undertaking pupillary assessment the following should be noted:

- any pre-existing irregularity with the pupils, e.g. cataracts, false eye and previous eye injury
- factors that cause pupillary dilation, e.g. medications, including tricyclics, atropine and sympathomimetics, and traumatic mydriasis (Bersten *et al.* 2003)
- factors that cause pupillary constriction, e.g. medications including narcotics (Fairley 2005) and topical beta blockers

Pupillary assessment should include the following observations:

- *Size* (millimetres): prior to shining light into the eyes, estimate pupil size using the scale printed on the neurological assessment chart as a comparison. The average size is 2–5 mm (Bersten *et al.* 2003). Both pupils should be equal in size.
- *Shape*: should be round; abnormal shapes may indicate cerebral damage; oval shape could indicate intracranial hypertension (Fairley 2005).
- *Reactivity to light*: a bright light source (usully a pen torch) should be moved from the outer aspect of the eye towards the pupil – a brisk pupil constriction should ensue. Following removal of the light source the pupil should return to its original size. The procedure should be repeated for the other eye. There should also be a consensual reaction to the light source, i.e. both eyes constrict when the light source is applied to the one. Unreactive pupils can be caused by an expanding mass, e.g. a blood clot exerting pressure on the third cranial nerve; a fixed and dilated pupil may be due to herniation of the medial temporal lobe (Bassett & Makin 2000). The reaction should be documented (Fig. 6.1) as + or B for brisk, – or 'N' for no reaction and sl or S for some or sluggish reaction (follow local policy). N.B. Lens implants or cataracts may prevent the pupil from constricting to light (Waterhouse 2005).
- *Equality*: both pupils should be the same shape, size and react equally to light.

PRINCIPLES OF INTRACRANIAL PRESSURE MONITORING

Intracranial pressure (ICP) is the pressure exerted by the normal cerebral components (brain tissue, blood and cerebrospinal fluid (CSF)) within the rigid structure of the skull. An increase in any one of these components means that the volume of the other is reduced by an equal amount (LeJeune & Howard-Fain 2002) to maintain homeostasis (Cree 2003). CSF is the most commonly displaced component and if ICP remains high after this is displaced cerebral blood volume is altered. When the maximal volume shift is reached further increases in intracranial volume will significantly increase ICP (LeJeune & Howard-Fain 2002). This can lead to a fall in cerebral perfusion pressure resulting in reduced cerebral perfusion and inadequate oxygen delivery.

Early detection of a raised ICP is therefore essential in order to prevent increasing cerebral damage and death. By inserting an ICP bolt or an intraventricular catheter, ICP can be continually monitored. The normal ICP is <10 mmHg; an ICP of >25 mmHg is a cause for concern, although cerebral perfusion pressure (CPP) is more important (Grant & Andrews 1999). The brain requires a cerebral perfusion pressure of >60 mmHg and a cerebral blood flow (CBF) of 50–100 ml to maintain optimum oxygenation (Cree 2003). CBF and CPP are directly related to mean arterial pressure (MAP) and ICP (Cree 2003):

$$CPP = MAP - ICP$$

Treatment is aimed at maintaining CPP.

Vital signs

It is important to monitor the patient's vital signs because they can be dramatically affected by a rise in ICP. The centres controlling heart rate, blood pressure, respiration and temperature are located in the brainstem. Of these four vital signs, the monitoring of respirations provides the clearest indication of cerebral function because they are controlled by different areas of the brain (Mallett & Dougherty 2000). The rate, character and pattern of respirations must be noted. Abnormal patterns in respirations have been discussed in Chapter 3.

A rising blood pressure and falling heart rate and respiratory rate are signs of raised ICP (Cushing's reflex) (Mooney & Comerford 2003). A sudden massive rise in ICP, e.g. following a large subarachnoid haemorrhage, can cause a Cheyne-Stokes breathing pattern (Shah 1999). Damage to the hypothalamus can cause changes in temperature.

Indications

Indications for ICP monitoring include:

- requirement for mechanical ventilation
- GCS score of <8: approximately two thirds of patients with head injuries with a GCS of 8 or less develop elevated ICP

- presence of small haematoma seen on the CT scan
- after decompression surgery

(Hinds & Watson 1996)

External ventricular drainage (EVD)

The use of EVDs is common in the management of severe traumatic brain injury, subarachnoid haemorrhage, tumours, CNS infections and acute shunt or ventricular obstruction (Littlejohns & Trimble 2005). In the operating theatre a catheter is introduced into the non-dominant ventricle through a burr hole and then tunnelled under the scalp and sutured (Woodward *et al*. 2002; Littlejohns & Trimble 2005). Connection to a transducer permits visible tracings on a monitor. In addition, the catheter is connected to a drainage system, allowing drainage by gravity if the ICP exceeds a set level, thus allowing nurses to maintain the pressure within normal parameters.

Maintaining accuracy

It is important to:

- Check all connections and tubing are secure (Woodward *et al*. 2002).
- Maintain the transducer at the same level as the foramen of Monro or at the level of the ear (Littlejohns & Trimble 2005).
- Record hourly the amount of CSF drained and empty (Woodward *et al*. 2002).
- Turn off before repositioning the patient and zero balance and recalibrate whenever the patient's position is altered (Woodward *et al*. 2002).
- Ensure air bubbles do not enter the transducer or tubing as this could dampen the trace and cause inaccurate ICP measurements (Littlejohns & Trimble 2005).

Suspected blockage of the drain must be reported to the neurosurgeon immediately (Woodward *et al*. 2002). Inaccurate or misleading measurements are the most common pitfalls encountered with ICP monitoring (Bergsneider & Becker 1995).

PRINCIPLES OF JUGULAR VENOUS BULB OXYGEN SATURATION MONITORING

This advanced form of monitoring is being increasingly used in neuroscience units, particularly for patients with head injuries. In combination with other clinical signs and physiological variables it enables the detection of cerebral ischaemia, provides a useful guide to more differentiated therapy and is prognostically accurate (Moore & Knowles 1999).

A fibreoptic catheter is inserted into the internal jugular vein and threaded upwards to the jugular bulb. Contraindications to insertion include significant trauma to the neck, a hypercoagulable state and bleeding diathesis (Moore & Knowles 1999).

Jugular venous bulb oxygen saturation monitoring (SjO_2) provides an indication of global cerebral oxygen delivery, but not regional ischaemia (Feldman & Robertson 1997). Cerebral oxygen consumption is usually 35–40% of available oxygen; the normal SjO_2 is therefore 60–65% (March 1994).

Changes in SjO_2 are reflective of changes in cerebral metabolic rate and cerebral blood flow (Woodrow 2000a). A reading below 50% for >15 minutes has been described as a jugular desaturation episode (Dearden 1991) and is associated with a poor neurological outcome (Gopinath *et al.* 1994). It should be noted that falls in SjO_2 can lag behind a rise in ICP and the clinical signs of deterioration (Sheinberg *et al.* 1992).

SjO_2 monitoring shares many of the problems encountered with pulse oximetry (Woodrow 2000a). Almost half of the apparent desaturation episodes are caused by technical problems, e.g. low light intensity (Sikes & Segal 1994). Light intensity should be monitored to ensure the accuracy of the readings.

Causes of high and low SjO_2

Causes of high SjO_2 (>80%) include:

- a rise in cerebral blood flow
- a fall in oxygen extraction
- raised ICP
- hyperventilation

(Sikes & Segal 1994)

Causes of low SjO_2 (<50%) include:

- hypoxia
- hypotension and cerebral hypoperfusion

High SjO_2 may reflect a fall in cerebral metabolic demand for oxygen, e.g. tissue death, hypothermia or the use of medications such as thiopentone; in fact an initial low SjO_2 followed by a gradual rise to >75% may be a preterminal event indicating initial ischaemia and then death of cerebral tissue (Moore & Knowles 1999).

PRINCIPLES OF MONITORING SEDATION

The purpose of sedation is to allow the patient to sleep undisturbed, minimise discomfort, abolish pain, reduce anxiety and facilitate organ–system support and nursing care (Bion & Oh 1997). An appropriate level of sedation produces a calm, cooperative patient who is easier to nurse and to treat (Gwinnutt 2006). Where possible the patient should still be able to communicate coherently, though in some situations, e.g. raised ICP, deeper sedation will be required. Midazolam and propofol are the most commonly used sedative drugs (Gwinnutt 2006).

Effects of over- and under-sedation

Over-sedation deprives the patient of life awareness and can cause respiratory and cardiovascular depression. Under-sedation exposes the patient to noxious stimuli, e.g. pain; increased protein breakdown from stress-induced hypermetabolism prolongs the process of weaning from the ventilator (Woodrow 2000a) resulting in prolonged bed rest, increasing the risk of immobility complications. Sedation should therefore be accurately assessed.

Assessment of sedation

It is difficult to assess sedation because the needs of patients vary (Shelly 1998) and discrepancies between practitioners' assessment exists (Westcott 1995). Haemodynamic changes are unreliable because most ICU patients are already labile (Shelly 1998). As corneal reflexes remain until the patient is in a deep coma, gently brushing the tips of the patient's eyelashes as a method of assessing whether the patient is sufficiently sedated to tolerate traumatic interventions, such as intubation, has been suggested (Woodrow 2000a).

Bion & Oh (1997) suggest the following methods of assessing sedation:

- *Level of consciousness* (or depth of sedation): to include any pain or discomfort, comprehension, tolerance of organ–system support and illness severity. There are various sedation scales currently in use, e.g. the Ramsey sedation scale (Ramsey *et al.* 1974) (Table 6.3).
- *Linear analogue scales*: when recorded by trained observers, these allow the various components of sedation to be measured independently. They are descriptively flexible and can be analysed either graphically or numerically (Wallace *et al.* 1988).

Problems associated with sedation

Problems associated with sedation include:

- hypotension
- prevention of sleep
- amnesia (Perrins *et al.* 1998)

Table 6.3 The Ramsey sedation scale.

Awake levels

(1) Patient anxious and agitated or restless or both
(2) Patient cooperative, orientated and tranquil
(3) Patient responds to command only

Asleep levels

(4) Brisk response
(5) Sluggish response
(6) No response

Source: Ramsey *et al.* 1974.

It is also important to be familiar with the specific side effects of the analgesics or hypnotics used for sedation.

MONITORING PAIN AND PAIN RELIEF

For the purpose of this book only some basic principles of monitoring pain and pain relief will be discussed. If the reader requires more in-depth information, there are books available that are dedicated to the subject of pain management, e.g. McCaffery and Beebe (1994).

Causes of pain

The patient may have acute pain, e.g. following surgery, or chronic pain, e.g. osteoarthritis. A post discharge survey of ICU patients carried out by Puntillo (1990) found that the following caused moderate to severe pain:

- surgery
- intubation
- removal of chest drains
- suction
- potassium infusions

In the critical care environment pain is aggravated by anxiety, fear, communication difficulties and the need for life-saving interventions (Adam & Osborne 1999).

Assessing pain

A barrier to effective pain management in the critically ill patient is a lack of systematic, comprehensive methods for assessing and treating pain (Puntillo *et al.* 2002). Frequently, the assessment of pain in critically ill patients can be difficult, particularly if they are intubated, sedated or have impaired psychomotor skills (Woodrow 2000a). The critically ill patient displays physiological variables, e.g. tachycardia, a rise in blood pressure, and physical responses, e.g. sweating and facial expression, which are particularly important (Adam & Osborne 1999) but can also be a sign of physiological problems rather than pain.

The use of pain assessment tools improves pain control (Puntillo *et al.* 2002), though unfortunately there is currently no ideal ICU pain assessment tool (Woodrow 2000a).

Relieving/preventing pain

The pioneering research carried out by Hayward (1975) demonstrated that preparation and honest explanations reduce pain, analgesia requirements and recovery time. Good communication is essential.

Methods of pain relief include analgesia (e.g. opiates), regional analgesia (e.g. epidurals) and nitrous oxide. Following administration of the chosen pain relief, it is important to evaluate its effectiveness. Although this should be common sense, nurses often fail to do this (Tittle & McMillan 1994). The use of a pain chart or of adequate recording in the patient's care plan is important if pain relief intervention is to be properly evaluated (Adam & Osborne 1999). It is also important to be alert to the possible side effects of pain relief, e.g. respiratory depression following opiate administration.

Epidural analgesia

Epidural analgesia is widely used postoperatively (Audit Commission 1997). A catheter is placed in the epidural space and analgesia (e.g. diamorphine, fentanyl) and an anaesthetic (e.g. 0.125% bupivacaine) can be administered either continuously through an infusion, by bolus injections, or patient-controlled bolus. The insertion site should be checked for leaks, signs of skin irritation and infection (Chapman & Day 2001). Close monitoring of the patient is essential to identify any complications which could include:

- respiratory depression
- hypotension
- nausea and vomiting
- pruritis
- urinary retention due to inhibition of the micturition reflex
- catheter migration
- meningitis (rare)

(Chapman & Day 2001)

The following parameters should be monitored:

- vital signs
- sedation score

- pain score
- fluid balance
- level/depth of block, e.g. using the Bromage score

(Hall 2000)

Scenario

A 25-year-old man is admitted to the Emergency Department with a head injury after falling off his bicycle. He is fully conscious, talking to you and there are no obvious injuries. What are your initial monitoring priorities?

The airway is clear and the neck is immobilised in a hard collar before cervical spinal injury can be excluded. BP 120/70 mmHg, respiratory rate 15/min, pulse 90/min, SpO$_2$ 98%, GCS 15; pupils are medium and both reacting equally and briskly to light. A CT scan is ordered. What ongoing monitoring will the patient require?

The patient's vital signs, SpO$_2$, GCS and pupillary assessment continue to be monitored. The patient starts to demonstrate signs of confusion. BP 120/75, pulse 94/min, SpO$_2$ 97%, GCS 13; pupils are medium and both reacting equally and briskly to light. What can be deduced from these observations?

The patient's vital signs are stable, but the slight drop in the GCS is of concern. The patient is taken for a CT scan. During the procedure his conscious level falls dramatically. BP 170/100, pulse 55, respiratory rate 10/min, SpO$_2$ 96%, GCS 9. He is responding and localising to pain and making incomprehensible sounds. His right pupil is dilated and not reacting to light. The left pupil is medium and reacting briskly to light. What can be deduced from these observations?

A right-sided subdural haematoma is confirmed by the CT scan. A rise in BP, fall in heart and respiratory rates and the deterioration in conscious level are signs consistent with a raised intracranial pressure. The unresponsive right pupil is consistent with third cranial nerve compression secondary to the right-sided subdural lesion. Urgent neurosurgical referral is required. Ongoing monitoring must continue with particular attention to the maintenance of a clear airway.

CONCLUSION

Monitoring neurological function is central to the care of all critically ill patients, particularly those with a head injury or other cerebral insult. It enables the early recognition and treatment of complications and can improve prognosis. It can also provide an indication to the function of other major systems in the body. The administration of medications, e.g. sedatives and paralysing agents, and any recent alcohol consumption should be taken into account.

REFERENCES

Adam, S. & Osborne, S. (1999) *Critical Care Nursing: Science and Practice*. Oxford Medical Publications, Oxford.

Albarran, J. & Price, T. (1998) *Managing the Nursing Priorities in Intensive Care*. Quay Books/Mark Allen Publishing, Dinton.

American College of Surgeons' Committee on Trauma (1997) *Student Course Manual*. American College of Surgeons, Chicago.

Aucken, S. & Crawford, B. (1998) Neurological assessment. In: D. Guerrero, ed. *Neuro-Oncology for Nurses*. Whurr Publishers, London.

Audit Commission (1997) *Anaesthesia Under Examination*. The Stationery Office, London.

Bassett, C. & Makin, L. (2000) eds. *Caring for the Seriously Ill Patient*. Arnold, London.

Bergsneider, M. & Becker, D. (1995) Intracranial pressure monitoring. In: S. Ayres, A. Grenvik, P. Holbrook & W. Shoemaker, eds. *Textbook of Critical Care* 3rd edn. W.B. Saunders, London.

Bersten, A.D., Soni, N. & Oh, T.E. (2003) *Oh's Intensive Care Manual* 5th edn. Butterworth-Heinman, London, UK.

Bion, J. & Oh, T. (1997) Sedation in intensive care. In: T. Oh, ed. *Intensive Care Manual* 4th edn. Butterworth Heinemann, Oxford.

Chapman, S. & Day, R. (2001) Spinal anatomy and the use of epidurals. *Professional Nurse* **16** (6), 1174–1177.

Cree, C. (2003) Aquired brain injury: acute management. *Nursing Standard* **18** (11), 45–54.

Dearden, N. (1991) Jugular venous oxygen saturation in the management of severe head injury. *Current Opinions in Anaesthesiology* **4**, 279–296.

Fairley, D. (2005) Using a coma scale to assess patient consciousness levels. *Nursing Times* **101** (25), 38–47.

Feldman, Z. & Robertson, C. (1997) Monitoring of cerebral haemodynamics with jugular bulb catheters. *Critical Care Clinics* **13** (1), 51–77.

Geraghty, M. (2005) Nursing the unconscious patient. *Nursing Standard* **20** (1), 54–64.

Gopinath, S., Robertson, C., Contant, C. *et al.* (1994) Jugular venous desaturation and outcome after head injury. *Journal of Neurological and Neurosurgical Psychiatry* **57**, 717–723.

Grant, I.S. & Andrews, P.J.D. (1999) ABC of Intensive Care Neurological Support. *British Medical Journal* **319**, 110–113.

Gwinnutt, C. (2006) *Clinical Anaesthesia* 2nd edn. Blackwell Publishing, Oxford.

Hall, J. (2000) Epidural analgesia management. *Nursing Times* **96** (28), 38–40.

Hayward, J. (1975) *Information: A Prescription Against Pain.* RCN, London.

Hinds, C.J. & Watson, D. (1996) *Intensive Care. A Concise Textbook*, 2nd edn. W.B. Saunders, London.

Holdgate, A. (2006) Variability in agreement between physicians and nurses when measuring the Glasgow Coma Scale in the emergency department limits its clinical usefulness. *Emergency Medicine Australasia* **18** (4), 379–384.

LeJeune, M. & Howard-Fain, T. (2002) Caring for patients with raised intracranial pressure. *Nursing* **32** (11), 32–34.

Littlejohns, L.R. & Trimble, B. (2005) Ask the experts. *Critical Care Nurse* **25** (3), 57–59.

Mallett, J. & Dougherty, L. (2000) eds. *The Royal Marsden Hospital Manual of Clinical Nursing Procedures.* Blackwell Science, Oxford.

March, K. (1994) Retrograde jugular catheter: monitoring SjO_2. *Journal of Neuroscience Nursing* **26** (1), 48–51.

McCaffery, M. & Beebe, A. (1994) *Pain: Clinical Manual for Nursing Practice.* C.V. Mosby, London.

McNarry, A.F. & Goldhill, D.R. (2004) Simple bedside assessment of level of consciousness: comparison of two simple assessment scales with the Glasgow Coma Scale. *Anaesthesia* **59**, 34–37.

Mooney, G.P. & Comerford, D.M. (2003) Neurological observations. *Nursing Times* **99** (17), 24–25.

Moore, P. & Knowles, M. (1999) Jugular venous bulb oxygen saturation monitoring in neuro critical care. *Care of the Critically Ill* **15** (5), 163–166.

Myburgh, E. & Oh, T. (1997) Disorders of consciousness. In: Oh T, ed. *Intensive Care Manual* 4th edn. Butterworth Heinemann, Oxford.

National Institute for Clinical Excellence (2003) *Head injury, triage, assessment, investigation and early management of head injury in infants, children and adults.* NICE, London.

Perrins, J., King, N. & Collings, J. (1998) Assessment of long-term psychological well-being following intensive care. *Intensive and Critical Care Nursing* **14** (3), 108–116.

Phillips, G. (1997) Pain relief in intensive care. In: T. Oh, ed. *Intensive Care Manual* 4th edn. Butterworth Heinemann, Oxford.

Price, T. (1996) An evaluation of neuro-assessment tools in the intensive care unit. *Nursing and Critical Care* **1** (2), 72–77.

Puntillo, K.A. (1990) Pain experiences of intensive care unit patients. *Heart and Lung* **19**, 526–533.

Puntillo, K., Stannard, D., Miaskowski, C. *et al.* (2002). Use of pain assessment and notation (P.A.I.N.) tool in critical care nursing practice: Nurses evaluation. *Heart Lung* **31**, 303–314.

Ramsey, M., Savage, T., Simpson, B. *et al.* (1974) Controlled sedation with alphaxalone and alphadolone. *British Medical Journal* **2**, 656–659.

Resuscitation Council UK (2006) *Advanced Life Support* 5th edn. Resuscitation Council UK, London.

Segatore, M. & Way, C. (1992) The Glasgow Coma Scale: time for change. *Heart Lung* **21** (6), 548–557.

Shah, S. (1999) Neurological assessment. *Nursing Standard* **13** (22), 49–54.

Sheinberg, M., Kanter, M., Robertson, C. *et al.* (1992) Continuous monitoring of jugular venous oxygen saturation in head injured patients. *Journal of Neurosurgery* **76**, 212–217.

Shelly, M. (1994) Assessing sedation. *Care of the Critically Ill* **10** (3), 118–121.

Shelly, M. (1998) Sedation in the ITU. *Care of the Critically Ill* **14** (3), 85–88.

Sheppard, M. & Wright, M. (2000) *High Dependency Nursing*. Ballière-Tindall, London.

Sikes, P. & Segal, J. (1994) Jugular venous bulb oxygen saturation monitoring for evaluating cerebral ischaemia. *Critical Care Nursing Quarterly* **17** (1), 9–20.

Silk, D. (1994) *Organisation of Nutritional Support in Hospitals*. BAPEN, London.

Smith, G. (2003) *ALERT Acute Life-Threatening Events Recognition and Treatment* 2nd edn. University of Portsmouth, Portsmouth.

Teasdale, G. & Jennett, B. (1974) Assessment of coma and impaired consciousness: a practical scale. *The Lancet* **2**, 81–84.

Tittle, M. & McMillan, S. (1994) Pain and pain-related side effects in an ICU and on a surgical unit: nurse's management. *American Journal of Critical Care* **3**, 25–30.

Wallace, P., Bion, J. & Ledingham, I. (1998) The changing face of sedative practice. In: I. Ledingham, ed. *Recent Advances in Critical Care Medicine*. Churchill Livingstone, Edinburgh.

Waterhouse, C. (2005) The Glasgow Coma Scale and other neurological observations. *Nursing Standard* **19** (33), 56–64.

Westcott, C. (1995) The sedation of patients in intensive care units. *Intensive and Critical Care Nursing* **11** (1), 26–31.

Woodrow, P. (2000a) *Intensive Care Nursing: A Framework for Practice*. Routledge, London.

Woodrow, P. (2000b) Head injuries: acute care. *Nursing Standard* **14** (35), 37–44.

Woodward, S. (1997) Neurological observations – Glasgow Coma Scale. *Nursing Times* **93** (45), Suppl 1–2.

Woodward, S., Addison, C., Shah, S. *et al.* (2002) Benchmarking best practice for external ventricular drainage. *British Journal of Nursing* **11** (1), 47–52.

Monitoring Renal Function | **7**

INTRODUCTION

Renal function should be closely monitored in all critically ill patients. First, it can provide an indication of the function of other systems, e.g. the cardiovascular system, where a low cardiac output will result in a diminished urine output. Nurses play a key role in the prevention and early detection of acute renal failure (ARF) (Redmond *et al.* 2004). The early recognition and prompt treatment of ARF are essential if prognosis is to be maximised. Patients receiving continuous renal replacement therapy (CRRT) is a frequent occurrence in ICU and these patients should also be closely monitored.

The aim of this chapter is to understand the principles of monitoring renal function.

LEARNING OBJECTIVES

At the end of the chapter the reader will be able to:

❏ describe the principles of *urinalysis*
❏ discuss the principles of *urine output monitoring*
❏ outline the key principles of monitoring *fluid balance*
❏ discuss the management of *acute renal failure*
❏ outline aspects of *management*
❏ outline the key aspects of *monitoring during renal replacement therapy*

PRINCIPLES OF URINALYSIS

Analysis of the volume, physical, chemical and microbiological properties of urine reveals much about the state of the body (Tortora & Grabowski 2003). Urinalysis can provide important information that can assist in diagnosis and can help in the monitoring of a patient's clinical condition. The purpose of urinalysis is three fold:

- *screening* for systemic disease, e.g. diabetes mellitus, renal conditions
- *diagnosis*: confirm or exclude suspected conditions e.g. urinary tract infections
- *management and planning*: to monitor the progress of an existing condition and/or plan programmes of care (Wilson 2005)

Appearance of urine

Normal urine is clear and pale yellow in appearance (Terrill 2002), but becomes turbid when left to stand. Variations in the appearance of urine include the following:

- *Pale*: urine is dilute; causes include overhydration, diabetes mellitus or insipidus and polyuria in renal disease resulting from the tubules failing to reabsorb water.
- *Dark*: urine is concentrated as seen in fluid depletion or contains urochrome pigment (breakdown of bile) (Tortora & Grabowski 2003).
- *Orange*: usually caused by specific drugs, e.g. rifampicin.
- *Pink/red*: may indicate haematuria, though other causes include ingestion of certain foodstuffs, e.g. beetroot.
- *Cloudy*: may indicate infection or the presence of red or white blood cells (Terrill 2002).
- *Debris*: may indicate infection.
- *Frothy*: may indicate significant proteinuria.

Odour

Normal, freshly voided urine is practically odourless. If left to stand for several hours it acquires a mild smell of ammonia (Tortora & Grabowski 2003). Infected urine has a 'fishy' smell (Rigby & Gray 2005). In diabetic patients with ketoacidosis or in patients who are anorexic or are not eating, acetone is excreted in the urine causing the urine to smell characteristically sweet.

Urinary incontinence

Urinary incontinence can occur transiently. Causes include urinary tract infections, delirium, excess urine output, e.g. following diuretics, faeces impaction and immobility (patient unable to reach the toilet or use a urinal) and spinal cord compression (necessitating emergency surgery).

Procedure for dipstick test of urine

A dipstick test of urine can accurately show the presence of a variety of substances, e.g. protein, glucose, ketones and blood, as well as the pH. To ensure reliable results, the following procedure for dipstick urine testing is recommended:

- Check the expiry date on the container, ensuring the testing strips are in date.
- Remove a testing strip from the container and replace the cap straight away.
- Dip the testing strip into a fresh sample of urine, ensuring all the reagent pads of the strip are covered. The urine must be fresh because 'stored' urine rapidly deteriorates which can cause false results (Dougherty & Lister 2004).
- Wipe off any excess urine on the rim of the specimen container.
- Place the testing strip flat on a dry surface to prevent the urine from running from square to square resulting in reagents mixing together. This may lead to an inaccurate result.
- Compare the reagent pads with the colour scale at time intervals stipulated by the manufacturer. If the strips are not read at exactly the time intervals specified, the reagents may not have had time to react which could cause inaccurate results (Dougherty & Lister 2004).
- Discard the urine sample and used testing strip.
- Record the results in the patient's notes and report any abnormalities.

It is essential to store and use the reagent strips correctly, following the manufacturer's recommendations, in order to ensure accurate and reliable results. The package insert supplied by the manufacturers will contain detailed instructions which normally include the following general points:

- The reagent strip should be stored in the container supplied by the manufacturer.
- The container cap should be replaced as soon as the reagent strip has been removed.
- The desiccant should never be removed from the bottle – some manufacturers incorporate it into the lid of the container so that it can not be lost.

- The container should be stored in a cool dry place, but not refrigerated.
- Reagent strips should not be used after the expiry date on the container.

Some drugs can influence urinalysis, e.g. high doses of aspirin or levodopa can cause a false negative reaction to glycosuria (Wilson 2005). It is therefore paramount to take into account the patient's medication when examining the results of dipstick urinalysis.

Best practice – urinalysis

Always use a fresh sample of urine collected in a clean, dry container
Observe sample for colour, appearance, smell and debris
Ensure reagent strip is in date
Ensure whole of reagent strip is immersed in urine sample
Wipe off excess urine, place horizontal and compare reagent pads with colour scale at time intervals stipulated by manufacturer and document results immediately
Safely discard strip and urine sample
Store reagent strips following manufacturer's recommendations

---

Significance of the results

Glycosuria is present when blood glucose is raised and the concentration of glucose in plasma exceeds the renal threshold (Wilson 2005) and can be associated with stress (Tortora & Grabowski 2003). Glycosuria can also occur in renal disease when the tubular threshold for glucose absorption has been altered (Terrill 2002). Urine tests are no longer recommended for diabetes control (Wilson 2005). If glycosuria is discovered a fasting blood glucose analysis is recommended.

Ketones (ketonuria) are produced during fat metabolism (Wilson 2005) and are suggestive of excessive fat breakdown as in starvation, fasting and uncontrolled diabetes mellitus (Stanley 2004).

Proteinuria is the presence of abnormally large quantities of protein, usually albumin (it is sometimes therefore termed albuminuria). Normally, no more than a trace of protein should be found in urine (250 mg protein in 24 hours), though sometimes a dipstick test may only show positive if the protein levels are 1.5 g or above in 24 hours. Proteinuria is indicative of an increase in membrane permeability due to injury or disease (Tortora & Grabowski 2003) and often a sign of renal compromise. Protein loss can be increased during febrile illness or after vigorous excercise

Persistent proteinuria is usually a sign of renal disease, e.g. urinary tract infection, pyelonephritis, or a renal complication of another disease, e.g. hypertension, congestive cardiac failure and pre-eclampsia. False-positive results can occur with alkaline urine and the use of disinfectants such as chlorhexidine.

The presence of blood (haematuria) is associated with diseases of the kidney or urinary tract, commonly infection, calculi, benign prostatatic hypertrophy, polycystic kidney, glomerular nephritis and tumours. Haematuria can also be caused by fractures of the pelvis and be present during menstruation (Wilson 2005). Dipstick urinalysis cannot distinguish red blood cells from myoglobin and haemoglobin therefore microscopic techniques are recommended to confirm the presence of blood cells (McDonald *et al.* 2006). The presence of haemoglobin (haemoglobinuria) is suggestive of a reaction to a blood transfusion, haemolytic anaemia or severe burns (Dougherty & Lister 2004). Reduction of sensitivity of the agent can occur if the patient is taking ascorbic acid or captopril (Wilson 2005).

Bilirubin is not normally detectable in urine (bilirubinuria) and its presence is usually indicative of liver or gall bladder disease, such as hepatitis, advanced cirrhosis, gallstones or carcinoma of the pancreas (Wilson 2005).

Urobilinogen presence in the urine is related to the production and conversion of bilirubin to urobilinogen in the gastrointestinal tract (Wilson 2005). Traces are normal but elevated levels may indicate haemolytic or pernicious anaemia, infectious hepatitis, biliary obstruction, jaundice, cirrhosis, congestive cardiac failure or infectious mononucleosis (Tortora & Grabowski 2003).

Nitrite is only found in urine in the presence of infection (Wilson 2005), as infective organisms convert nitrate to nitrite. A negative result does not exclude the presence of infection.

False-positive results can occur in patients taking vitamin C (Rigby & Gray 2005).

Leucocytes in urine (pyuria) usually indicates inflammation or infection (Terrill 2002) and is an indication for laboratory testing. False-negative results can be caused by glycosuria and drugs such as nitrofurantoin and rifampicin (Rigby & Gray 2005).

The normal range of urine pH is 6.4–8.0 (average is 7.0) (Tortora & Grabowski 2003). Urine pH is an indicator of the degree of hydrogen ion secretion and the reabsorption of bicarbonate ions (Terrill 2002). Acidic urine (pH < 7.0) is found in patients with diabetic ketoacidosis, starvation, high-protein diet and potassium depletion. Alkaline urine (pH > 7.0) may be indicative of urinary tract infection, or be caused by vomiting or excessive intake of antacids (Wilson 2005), vegetarian diets, citrus fruits and dairy products (Tortora & Grabowski 2003).

The specific gravity of urine is a measure of urine osmolality (Redmond *et al*. 2004), the normal range being 1.001–1.035. Urine of high specific gravity is concentrated and a urine with a low specific gravity is dilute (Terrill 2002). High values are indicative of dehydration and low values are found with high fluid intake, diabetes insipidus, renal failure, hypercalcaemia or hypokalaemia (Wilson 2005).

Other urine tests

Osmolality
Osmolality is the number of particles of solute per kilogram of water (Tortora & Grabowski 2003) and is a measure of the kidney's ability to concentrate urine (Terrill 2002).

Creatinine clearance
Creatinine clearance is the standard test to assess glomerular function. The principle of clearance is that an estimation of a known substance (which is only excreted in the urine) in the plasma is compared with the amount in the urine. Creatinine is produced by the breakdown of creatinine phosphate, which is manufactured by the muscle mass at a fairly constant rate. It is present in the circulation and is filtered by the glomeruli.

Microscopy and culture
Being the most concentrated, the first voided urine of the day is the best for culture. Ideally the sample should be taken before starting a broad-spectrum antibiotic, which may be given in the interim period before a specific sensitivity is identified.

URINE OUTPUT MONITORING
Although urine output is only an index to renal perfusion, it is frequently used as a guide to the adequacy of cardiac output (renal perfusion amounts to 25% of the cardiac output). However the use of diuretics, such as frusemide or dopamine, abolishes its value as a haemodynamic monitor (Gomersall & Oh 1997).

Urine is composed of 95% water and 5% solids, mainly urea and sodium chloride; it is slightly acidic (pH 6.0) and has a specific gravity of 1.010–1.030 (SG of water is 1.000) (Wilson 2005). The average urine output in a healthy adult is 1000–1500 ml per day. Listed below are the generally accepted rates of urine production associated with urinary output disorders:

- anuria: <50 ml of urine in 24 hours
- oliguria: <400 ml of urine in 24 hours
- polyuria: >3000 ml of urine in 24 hours
- dysuria: painful micturition

(Tortora & Grabowski 2003).

All critically ill patients will require a urinary catheter. If urine output measurements are required the patient should be catheterised and an hourly urine drainage bag attached (Fig. 7.1). The urinary catheter should be closely monitored because it can become blocked, e.g. from a blood clot, or become occluded, e.g. due to kinking. If an assessment of bladder volume is required, bedside bladder scanning is now widely available for nurses to use. Sometimes bladder washouts are indicated if difficulties with drainage are encountered, e.g. if there is a lot of debris or blood clots in the urine.

MONITORING FLUID BALANCE
Monitoring fluid balance in the critically ill patient is paramount. Physiological mechanisms, disease processes and treatment side effects are just a few of the numerous factors that can affect fluid

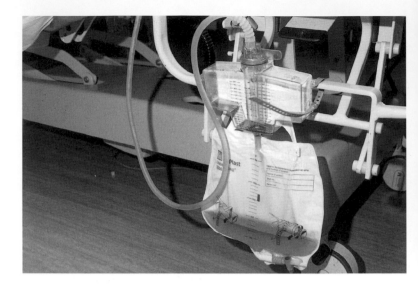

Fig. 7.1 Hourly urine drainage bag.

status (Sheppard & Wright 2000). Fluid and electrolyte overload is sometimes difficult to avoid and is commonly found in patients with multi-organ failure (Gosling 1999).

Careful monitoring of the fluid balance chart must be maintained and this should include all input and output. Monitoring the patient for signs of fluid loss/gain should also be undertaken and Table 7.1 provides an overview of this. The importance of monitoring urine output, urine osmolality and specific gravity of urine have already been discussed.

Daily measurement of serum sodium, potassium, urea and creatinine together with 24-hour urine volume are required to assess fluid and electrolyte balance. In addition, fluid balance charts from the preceding few days should be compared to serum and urine urea and electrolyte values. This will help evaluate the patient's response to fluid administration and will guide the fluid regime over the next 12–24 hours (Gosling 1999). The nature and

Table 7.1 Systemic signs and symptoms of fluid loss and gain.

System	Signs in fluid loss	Signs in fluid gain	Monitoring and nursing observation
Cardiovascular	Increase heart rate Irregular thready pulse Reduced blood pressure and CVP	Increased heart rate, BP, CVP Neck vein distension may be evident	Pulse Blood pressure CVP
Respiratory	Increased respiratory rate Hyperventilation	Increased rate Dyspnoea and pulmonary oedema may be evident	Nature and frequency of respirations Signs of waterlogging of pulmonary circulation Oxygenation status – skin colour Saturation, i.e. pulse oximetry/blood gases
Urinary system	Urine output decreased, or increased in diabetes insipidus	Output may be increased or decreased depending on the underlying cause and renal function	Volume of urine output/24-hour period
General orientation	Apprehension Restlessness	Confusion Irritability	General orientation status
Skin	Texture is dry and lax, under-perfusion of tissues and reduced vascularity leading to skin colour change, dry mucous membranes and evidence of thirst Excessive perspiration accompanies increased body temperature	Dependent, generalised and/or pitting oedema The skin may be warm, moist and swollen with the appearance of being tight and shiny	General appearance/hydrational status Colour Temperature Condition of mucous membranes

Reprinted by permission of Baillière Tindall from Sheppard & Wright (2000).

volume of any fluid replacement therapy will depend on fluid loss (Sheppard & Wright 2000).

MANAGEMENT OF ACUTE RENAL FAILURE (ARF)

ARF is a syndrome characterised by a rapid (hours to days) decrease in the kidney's ability to eliminate waste products which results in an accumulation of end products of nitrogen metabolism (urea and creatinine) (Bersten *et al.* 2003).

Inadequate renal perfusion resulting from a serious insult, e.g. haemorrhage, burns, sepsis or trauma, which has resulted in circulatory shock, is the commonest cause of ARF on the intensive care unit (Bellomo 1997; Hamilton 1999). However, ARF can be attributed to a multiplicity of different diseases and pathophysiological mechanisms. ARF can often be prevented if the predisposing factors are recognised and treated promptly (Redmond *et al.* 2004).

ARF can be classified into three groups:

- *Pre-renal*: caused by inadequate renal perfusion; causes include a significant fall in cardiac output, severe hypotension and intravascular volume depletion, e.g. haemorrhagic or septic shock, peritonitis and pancreatitis. This form of ARF is most commonly seen on the ICU (Bersten *et al.* 2003).
- *Intrinsic (parenchymal)*: occurs when there is structural damage to the renal parenchyma such as acute tubular necrosis (ATN). ATN occurs because of sustained renal hypoperfusion (Perkins & Kisiel 2005). Causes include; coagulopathies, vasculitis, nephrotoxins and acute interstitial nephritis (Terrill 2002). Intrinsic renal failure differs from pre-renal failure in that correcting the cause does not guarantee the return of full function (Terrill 2002).
- *Post-renal*: caused by obstruction of urine drainage either above or below the bladder (Redmond *et al.* 2004). Causes include: prostatic hypertrophy, renal calculi, carcinoma of the cervix and tumours.

In all cases, particularly if the patient has persistent anuria or intermittent anuria, it is important to exclude bladder outflow obstruction: this possibility should be suspected in patients who have previously had prostate enlargement or who have had trauma or recent surgery to the pelvic area (Hinds & Watson 1996). In addition, if the patient is catheterised it is important to exclude a blocked catheter.

Diagnosis

The clinical presentation of ARF despite adequate resuscitation:

- anuria or profound oliguria
- progressive rise in blood creatinine and urea levels
- developing metabolic acidosis
- rising serum potassium and phosphate levels
- multi-organ dysfunction is common

Once bladder outflow obstruction has been excluded it is important to establish whether the patient is in pre-renal, intrinsic or post-renal failure (Hinds & Watson 1996).

Clinical course

The clinical course of ARF can be classified into three distinct phases (Redmond *et al*. 2004):

- *Oliguric/non-oliguric phase*: in the oliguric phase the total urine output is <400 ml in 24 hours. The non-oliguric phase can usually be associated with nephrotoxic agents and although urine output may not be reduced, the ability to produce a concentrated urine is severely impaired causing a drop in solute excretion (Redmond *et al*. 2004; Perkins & Kisiel 2005).
- *Diuretic phase*: this is marked by increased urine output, sometimes 3000 ml in 24 hours. It is essential to maintain hydration and accurate fluid and electrolyte balance during this phase. The prognosis depends on its severity and whether the patient is critically ill.
- *Recovery phase*: tubular function is restored, diuresis subsides and the kidneys begin to function normally again.

The mortality rate for patients with ARF remains high despite recent advances in treatment modalities (Dirkes 2000; Terrill 2002; Bellomo *et al*. 2004). This is primarily because ARF is often accompanied by other organ failure and is estimated to be 40–80% dependent on case mix.

Prevention of ARF

Due to the poor prognosis, prevention of ARF in the critically ill patient is paramount. It is important to be able to recognise the early signs of impaired renal function; provided chronic renal failure is prevented, recovery of renal tissue (unlike other major organs) is usually complete (Woodrow 2000). Redmond *et al.* (2004) suggest the following to attempt to prevent ARF:

- early identification of those patients at risk
- accurate recording of fluid balance
- accurate recording and interpretation of physiological observations
- nutritional support to prevent malnutrition
- aggressive fluid resuscitation where indicated
- avoidance of nephrotoxic drugs

Complications of ARF

Hyperkalaemia is the most serious electrolyte imbalance seen in ARF (Bellomo 1997). Characteristic ECG changes include elevated and pointed T waves. Cardiac arrhythmias and cardiac arrest may ensue and active treatment is normally required, e.g. calcium resonium, insulin (and dextrose), renal replacement therapy and, in extreme situations, intravenous calcium chloride. Continuous cardiac monitoring is essential to ensure early detection of cardiac arrhythmias.

Patients with ARF are immunosupressed because of uraemia (Perkins & Kisiel 2005) and are therefore at greater risk of developing infections such as pneumonia, urinary tract infection (UTI), wound infection and sepsis (Redmond *et al.* 2004).

Adequate nutritional support is required. A critically ill patient with ARF should receive aggressive, protein-rich nutritional support, either enterally or parenterally; calorie requirements are no different to those of other ICU patients without ARF (Bellomo *et al.* 1991). Potassium, sodium and fluid intake should be restricted. Close monitoring of blood glucose levels is essential, particularly if the patient is on dietary supplements.

The patient who is in the oliguric phase of ARF requires careful fluid balance assessment. To prevent volume overload, a general working rule is the previous day's urine output plus 500 ml for insensible loss. Consideration must be given to such variables as pyrexia, diarrhoea and wound drainage.

Serial weights may be more reliable than fluid balance assessment but are not widely used due to technical difficulties; rapid daily gains and losses in weight are usually related to changes in fluid volume. It is also important to observe for signs of fluid overload, e.g. raised CVP, generalised oedema, pulmonary oedema and dyspnoea.

Clinical features of uraemia include nausea, vomiting, hiccoughs, confusion, irritability, altered conscious level, infection and bleeding. It is important to observe for these complications and treat appropriately.

Criteria for the initiation of CRRT:

- oliguria (urine output: <200 ml/12 hours)
- anuria (urine output 0–50 ml/12 hours)
- urea >35 mmol/l
- creatinine >400 μmol/l
- K^+ >6.5 mmol/l or rapidly rising
- pulmonary oedema unresponsive to diuretics
- uncompensated metabolic acisosis (pH < 7.1)
- Na <110 and >160 mmol/l
- temperature >40°C
- uraemic complications (encephalopathy, neuropathy, pericarditis)
- overdose with a dialysable toxin

If two of the above criteria are met, CRRT is strongly recommended (Bersten *et al.* 2003).

MONITORING DURING CONTINUOUS RENAL REPLACEMENT THERAPY

CRRT in ICU is an extracorporeal venous system whereby blood is driven through a haemofilter to remove water, electrolytes, small- and medium-sized molecules from the blood via diffusion, osmosis and convection (Dirkes 2000) (Fig. 7.2). To maximise the removal of solutes dialysate fluid is added to the circuit which flows around the fibres of the filter.

CRRT has many modalities:

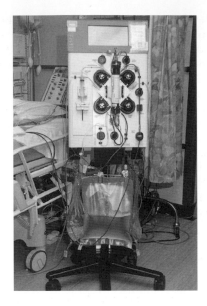

Fig. 7.2 Continuous renal replacement therapy.

- *Continuous venovenous haemofiltration (CVVH)*: blood is driven through the semi-permeable membrane filter and replacement fluid is added to prevent excessive loss of fluid. Solutes are mainly removed by convection.
- *Slow continuous ultrafiltration (SCUF)*: Blood is driven through the semi-permeable membrane filter but there is no fluid replacement. SCUF is utilised for fluid removal in fluid overload, as solute clearance is very low.
- *Continuous venovenous haemodialysis (CVVHD)*: Blood is driven through the semi-permeable membrane filter with the addition of a countercurrent dialysate solution to improve solute clearance. Replacement fluid is not administered.
- *Continuous venovenous haemodiafiltration (CVVHDF)*: CVVHDF is the same principle as CVVHD but with the addition of replacement fluid to balance fluid losses. This is the most frequently used modality in the ICU patient with ARF.

Blood biochemistry, a full blood count and clotting profile are taken as a screening prior to the procedure to provide a baseline. To facilitate patient monitoring pulse oximetry is used.

ECG monitoring is necessary, as cardiac arrhythmias can occur, particularly if hypokalaemia is present. Hypotension will occur if the rate of fluid being removed in the dialyser exceeds the plasma refilling rate in the patient, so haemodynamic measurements are also required. In addition, during the first 2 hours of therapy, a sudden drop in blood pressure can occur following fluid drainage (Dougherty & Lister 2004).

A strict fluid balance must be maintained to prevent accidental hypovolaemia and hypervolaemia, and a careful watch kept on the patient's temperature as circulating the blood outside the body may precipitate hypothermia. Pyrexia may indicate infection.

Circuit pressure monitoring is also important – a rise may indicate clotting of the line or filter. The patient's coagulation status must be closely monitored: anticoagulation of the circuit is often required and the patient is therefore at risk of haemorrhage, so any signs of bleeding from vascular access sites, mucous membranes, gastrointestinal tract, etc. should be noted. As the blood circulates ensure the bubble trap fluid remains constant.

Complications of haemodialysis and haemofiltration

These include the following:

- *Haemolysis*, resulting from damage to red blood cells as they pass through the pump, can lead to hyperkalaemia and cardiac arrest. Observe for chest pain and dyspnoea. Blood in the venous circuit may have the appearance of 'port wine' (Adam & Osborne 1999).
- *Air embolism*: observe for chest pain and dyspnoea.
- *Reaction to the membrane*: if a cellulose-based cuprophane (dialyser membrane) is used, it may cause a systematic inflammatory response syndrome (Hakim 1993) which can lead to delayed renal recovery and increased mortality (Hakim *et al.* 1994).
- *Disequilibrium*: this is caused by a sudden removal of urea and uraemic toxins and the patient can present with headache,

vomiting, restlessness, convulsions and coma (Adam & Osborne 1999).

- *Infection*: strict attention must be paid to maintaining aseptic conditions at all times.

Scenario

Donald was admitted to the ICU after blunt abdominal trauma sustained in an industrial accident. He was ventilated following a diagnostic laparotomy and repair of mesenteric tear. He was progressing steadily over the next 24 hours when his condition suddenly deteriorated. He developed cardiovascular instability and required inotropic support. He was hyperpyrexic with a white cell blood count of 27.8 cells/l. Intra-abdominal sepsis was suspected.

He was taken to theatre for a further laparotomy to ascertain the focus of the suspected sepsis. At operation haemorrhagic pancreatitis was diagnosed and several irrigation drains were inserted into the abdomen and saline irrigation commenced. After return to the unit his condition deteriorated with inotropic requirements increasing and oliguria developing. It was confirmed that the urinary catheter was not blocked or kinked. Diuretics were administered without effect and anuria developed. The patient's blood chemistry was:

Potassium: 6.8 mmol/l
Serum urea: 29 mg/dl
Creatinine: 420 mg/dl

A diagnosis of acute tubular necrosis (ATN) was made. What is the most appropriate treatment?

Continuous renal replacement therapy is the only treatment suitable for Donald in this scenario.

Haemofiltration was established without complications, removal rate of 120 ml/h, using heparin as the anticoagulant in the circuit. Initially blood was taken twice daily for biochemical analysis to ascertain the efficacy of the CRRT in the reduction of serum creatinine and urea and maintenance of normal potassium levels.

Haemofiltration continued for a further 10 days during which time inotropic requirements reduced and renal function returned to normal. The patient made a full recovery from this episode of ATN secondary to sepsis.

CONCLUSION

Monitoring renal function is central to the care of a critically ill patient. It can provide an indication of the function of the kidneys as well as the performance of other major systems of the body. The early recognition and prompt treatment of acute renal failure is essential if prognosis is to be maximised.

REFERENCES

Adam, S. & Osborne, S. (1999) *Critical Care Nursing: Science and Practice*. Oxford Medical Publications, Oxford.

Bellomo, R., Martin, H., Parkinn, G. *et al*. (1991) Continuous arteriovenous haemodiafiltration in the critically ill; influence on major nutrient balance. *Intensive Care Medicine* **17**, 399–402.

Bellomo, R. (1997) Acute renal failure. In: T.E. Oh, ed. *Intensive Care Manual* 4th edn. Butterworth Heinemann, Oxford.

Bellomo, R., Ronco, C., Kellum, J.A. *et al*. (2004) Acute renal failure – definition, outcome measures, animal models, fluid therapy and information technology needs. Critical Care **8**, R204–212.

Bersten, A.D., Soni, N. & Oh, T.E. (2003) *Oh's Intensive Care Manual*. Butterworth-Heinemann, Philadelphia.

Corwin, H.L. & Bonventre, J.V. (1989) Factors influencing survival in acute renal failure. *Seminars in Dialysis* **2**, 220–225.

Dirkes, S.M. (2000) Continuous renal replacement therapy: dialytic therapy for acute renal therapy in intensive care. *Nephrology Nursing Journal* **27** (6), 581–592.

Dougherty, L. & Lister, S. (2004) *The Royal Marsden Hospital Manual of Clinical Nursing Procedures* 6th edn. Blackwell Publishing, Oxford.

Gokal, R., Ash, S., Holfrich, B. *et al*. (1993) Peritoneal catheters and exit site practices: toward optimum peritoneal access. *Peritoneal Dialysis International* **13**, 29–39.

Gomersall, C. & Oh, T. (1997) Haemodynamic monitoring. In: T. Oh, ed. *Intensive Care Manual* 4th edn. Butterworth Heinemann, Oxford.

Gosling, P. (1999) Fluid balance in the critically ill: the sodium and water audit. *Care of the Critically Ill* **15** (1), 11–18.

Hakim, R. (1993) Clinical implications of hemodialysis membrane biocompatability. *Kidney International* **44**, 484–494.

Hakim, R., Wingard, R. & Parker, R. (1994) Effect of dialysis membrane in the treatment of patients with acute renal failure. *New England Journal of Medicine* **331**, 1338–1342.

Hamilton, M. (1999) Cause and effects of renal failure. *Nursing Times* **95** (12), 59–60.

Hinds, C.J. & Watson, D. (1996) *Intensive Care: A concise textbook* 2nd edn. W.B. Saunders, London.

Khanna, R., Nolph, K. & Oreopoulos, D. eds (1993) Complications during peritoneal dialysis. In: *The Essentials of Peritoneal Dialysis.* Kluwer Academic, Dordrecht.

King, B. (1995) Acute renal failure. *Registered Nurse* March, 35–39.

Lohr, J.W., McFarlane, M.J. & Grantham, A.J. (1988) A clinical index to predict survival in acute renal failure patients requiring dialysis. *American Journal of Kidney Disease* **11**, 254–259.

Luzar, M. (1991) Exit site infection in CAPD: a review. *Peritoneal Dialysis International* **11**, 333–340.

McDonald, M.M., Swagerty, M.D. & Wetzel, L. (2006) Assessment of microscopic haematuria in adults. *American Family Physician* **73**, 1748–1754.

McMurray, S.D., Luft, F.C., Maxwell, D.R. *et al.* (1978) Prevailing patterns and predictor variables in patients with acute tubular necrosis. *Archives of Internal Medicine* **138**, 950–955.

Perkins, C. & Kisiel, M. (2005) Utilising physiological knowledge to care for acute renal failure. *British Journal of Nursing* **14** (14), 768–773.

Redmond, A., McDevitt, M. & Barnes, S. (2004) Acute renal failure: recognition and treatment in ward patients. *Nursing Standard* **18** (22), 46–53.

Rigby, D. & Gray, K. (2005) Understanding urine testing. *Nursing Times* **101** (12), 60–62.

Sheppard, M. (2000) Monitoring fluid balance in acutely ill patients. *Nursing Times* **96** (21), 39–40.

Sheppard, M. & Wright, M. (2000) *High Dependency Nursing* 1st edn, p. 249. Baillière Tindall, London.

Spiegel, D.M., Ullian, M.E., Zerbe, G.O. & Berl, T. (1991) Determinants of survival and recovery in acute renal failure patients dialysed in intensive care units. *American Journal of Nephrology* **11**, 44–47.

Stanley, K. (2004) Urine testing. *Diabetes Forecast* RG64–RG69.

Terrill, B. (2002) *Renal Nursing – a practical approach*. Ausmed Publications, Victoria, Australia.

Torrance, C. & Elley, K. (1997) Respiration, technique and observation 1. *Nursing Times* **93** (43), Suppl. 1–2.

Tortora, G.J. & Grabowski, S.R. (2003) *Principles of Anatomy and Physiology* 10th edn. John Wiley & Sons Inc, New Jersey, USA.

Wilson, L.A. (2005) Urinalysis. *Nursing Standard* **19** (35), 51–54.

Woodrow, P. (2000) *Intensive Care Nursing, a Framework for Practice*. Routledge, London.

Monitoring Gastrointestinal Function

8

INTRODUCTION

The importance of the gastrointestinal (GI) tract as a defence system and as an essential resource for other organs is increasingly being recognised. The support of its functions is now considered an essential part of the global treatment of a critically ill patient (Adam & Osborne 2005). It is therefore essential to be able to monitor GI function accurately.

The aim of this chapter is to understand the principles of monitoring GI function.

LEARNING OBJECTIVES

At the end of the chapter the reader will be able to:

❏ describe the assessment of *bowel function*
❏ discuss the significance of *nausea and vomiting*
❏ discuss the monitoring of *stomas and fistulas*
❏ outline the causes of acute *upper gastrointestinal bleeding*
❏ outline the assessment of *intestinal obstruction*
❏ discuss the principles of monitoring *pancreatic function*

ASSESSMENT OF BOWEL FUNCTION

Assessing bowel function can provide important information that can assist in diagnosis and can help in the monitoring of a patient's clinical condition. The following should be noted:

• *patient's normal bowel activity*: frequency of bowel movement and any unexplained changes in bowel habit
• *consistency of the faeces*: hard, bulky or pellet-like suggestive of constipation; loose, watery and frequent faeces are suggestive of diarrhoea
• *colour of faeces*: normal faeces should be brown due to the presence of modified bowel pigments (Bruce & Finley 1997); dark

In all cases of nausea and vomiting the following are important:

- the patient's medical history and present condition
- examination of the patient's abdomen to determine whether there is pain, tenderness, guarding, presence of bowel sounds
- the patient's medication regime, both past and current
- blood biochemical assessment
- a rectal examination
- a plain abdominal radiograph

(Bruce & Finley 1997).

The timing of vomiting together with the volume and consistency of the vomit are also helpful.

Timing of vomiting
Vomiting that occurs more than an hour after eating is characteristic of obstruction of the gastric outlet, while early morning vomiting is typical of pregnancy, alcoholism and raised intracranial pressure (Talley & O'Connor 1998).

Volume of vomit
The volume of the vomit is important: a large volume may be indicative of gastric outflow obstruction. If there are small amounts of vomit it is important to ensure that the patient is actually vomiting and not just expectorating – the litmus paper test is recommended.

Consistency of vomit
The consistency is important:

- *'coffee-grounds'*: old blood clots in vomit; can also be caused by iron tablets, red wine and, of course, coffee ingestion
- *fresh blood*: the presence of fresh blood is indicative of bleeding from the upper gastrointestinal tract
- *yellow/green*: presence of bile and upper small bowel contents is suggestive of obstruction
- *faeculent*: brown offensive material from the small bowel, a late sign of small intestinal obstruction (Talley & O'Connor 1998)
- *projectile*: causes include pyloric stenosis and raised intracranial pressure

MONITORING STOMAS AND FISTULAS

Stomas

Several factors can influence the characteristics of output from stomas including medication, diet and amount of bowel removed. The position of the stoma is also significant: basically the more proximal the stoma, the more fluid the effluent and the more caustic its effect on the skin due to the presence of chemical irritants effluent from the stoma (Rolstad & Erwin-Toth 2004). In addition to chemical irritants, other causes of loss of skin integrity include stripping off the ostomy bag adhesive, infection, allergy to the stoma bag adhesive and underlying skin disease, e.g. eczema (Rolstad & Erwin-Toth 2004).

The skin surrounding the stoma should be closely observed for early signs of maceration (Myers 1998; Herlufsen *et al*. 2006). Documentation of the size, length and colour should be regularly undertaken and output from the stoma should be recorded.

Fistulas

An enterocutaneous fistula is an abnormal communication between a section of the gastrointestinal tract and the skin (Renton *et al*. 2006). It usually arises from the small or large intestine, from an underlying area of diseased bowel or as a complication of abdominal surgery (Hollington *et al*. 2004). It can lead to a life-threatening deterioration in the patient's condition with sepsis, electrolyte disturbances, malnutrition and dehydration (Rinsema 1994). The location of the fistula along the bowel will determine the type of effluent produced, e.g. a small bowel fistula can lead to the leaking of copious volumes of corrosive fluid (Renton *et al*. 2006). Monitoring priorities include recording the consistency and volume of the effluent and observing the surrounding skin for maceration. Monitoring skin integrity is a key priority (Renton *et al*. 2006).

ACUTE UPPER GASTROINTESTINAL BLEEDING

Acute upper gastrointestinal bleeding is a common admission to the ICU and is a major cause of morbidity and mortality. It has a 10% mortality rate (Morris 1992). Peptic ulcer and varices are the two most frequent causes of upper GI bleeding (Fiore *et al*. 2005).

GI bleeding usually manifests itself through haematemesis and melaena or more dangerously through an enlarged abdomen with associated abdominal pain. The vomit may either be bright red or coffee-ground in appearance, depending on the length of time the blood has been in contact with gastric secretions (gastric acid converts bright red haemoglobin to brown haematin) and on the amount of gastric contents at the time of the bleeding (Hudak *et al.* 1998). A history of vomiting and retching preceding the GI bleeding suggests Mallory-Weiss syndrome – a tear at the junction of the stomach and the oesophagus secondary to forceful vomiting/coughing.

Although most GI bleeds stop spontaneously, approximately 20% will re-bleed in hospital and many of these will need surgical intervention. Surgery remains the most definitive intervention to stop bleeding. Upper GI bleeds are commonly seen in the ICU or high dependency unit (HDU) because of the vast blood supply to the stomach and oesophagus. Bleeding is therefore more likely to be severe causing haemodynamic instability requiring massive fluid resuscitation.

Monitoring priorities include:

- assessing for signs of hypovolaemia and shock
- estimating blood loss and accurate maintenance of fluid balance
- determining the cause of the bleed if possible (Table 8.2)

Table 8.2 Causes of upper gastrointestinal bleeding.

Frequency	Causes
Common	Duodenal and gastric ulceration; oesophagitis; gastritis; duodenitis; varices; Mallory–Weiss tear
Less common	Carcinomas; bleeding diathesis; leiomyomas; aortic aneurysm fistula
Rare (less than 1%)	Dieulafoy lesion; angiomas; hereditary haemorrhagic telangiectasia; pseudoxanthoma elasticum; Ehlers–Danlos syndrome; haemobilia; pancreatic bleeding; foreign body

Reprinted from *Nursing in Gastroenterology*, Bruce and Finlay, © 1997, with permission from Elsevier Ltd.

- monitoring fluid balance
- monitoring the function of other major systems
- laboratory investigations, e.g. full blood count (FBC), pro-thrombin time, liver function tests (LFTs), platelet count, urea and electrolytes (U+Es)
- monitoring intra-abdominal pressures for signs of increasing pressure

If the GI bleed is due to leaking oesophageal varices a Seng-staken tube may be helpful to apply pressure on the bleeding points. Close monitoring of tube position together with the patient's airway and respiratory status is important.

ASSESSMENT OF INTESTINAL OBSTRUCTION
Intestinal obstruction can occur in either the small or large bowel. It can lead to bowel strangulation, infarction and perforation, resulting in potentially life-threatening peritoneal and systemic infection (Hudak *et al.* 1998). It can be classified as mechanical or non-mechanical. Mechanical obstruction results from a physical blockage of the intestinal lumen which may be complete or incomplete. Causes include adhesions, malignancy, hernias, bolus obstruction and bowel strangulation, e.g. volvulus. Non-mechanical obstruction is caused by ineffective intestinal peristalsis (par-alytic ileus), causes of which include trauma, handling of the bowel during surgery, peritonitis and electrolyte imbalance (Hudak *et al.* 1998).

Detailed below are the key monitoring considerations:

- *blood pressure* and *pulse measurements* to detect early signs of shock
- *temperature* – pyrexia is usually present, though does not nor-mally exceed 37.8°C (Hudak *et al.* 1998)
- *abdominal girth measurements*: abdominal distension is a key clinical feature
- *vomiting*: the higher the obstruction, the more profuse the vomit
- *fluid and electrolyte balance*
- *abdominal pain*: characteristics and severity
- *bowel function*: consistency of faeces, regularity, volume

PRINCIPLES OF MONITORING PANCREATIC FUNCTION

The pancreas secretes water to dilute chyme, bicarbonate to neutralise postgastric chyme and enzymes to help with digestion. Its endocrine function is discussed in Chapter 10.

Acute pancreatitis, which is associated with significant morbidity and mortality rates (Steinberg & Tenner 1994; Felderbauer *et al*. 2005), is commonly caused by long-term alcohol abuse and gall bladder disease, which account for over 75% of cases (Adam & Osborne 2005). Pancreatitis can compromise most of the major systems in the body. Therefore close monitoring is required. The key priorities are listed below:

- *Haemodynamic monitoring*: hypovolaemia and fluid volume imbalances may be present (large volumes of fluid can leak into extravascular spaces).
- *Pulse oximetry and arterial blood gas analysis*: respiratory failure can be a complication.
- *ECG monitoring*: electrolyte imbalances can cause arrhythmias.
- *Blood sugar estimations*: hyperglycaemia may occur as a result of impaired insulin production and increased release of glucagon.
- *Temperature*: the main cause of pyrexia is hypermetabolism, though infection may also be the cause (Woodrow 2000).
- *Nutritional status*: patient will be nil by mouth, parenteral nutrition will probably be started (Robin *et al*. 1990; Pandol 2006). If there is long-term alcohol abuse, nutrition is an even greater priority.
- *Serum amylase*: usually increases up to tenfold within 6 hours (Reece-Smith 1997).
- *Pain*: the patient may have severe abdominal pain.

Scenario

William, a 48-year-old man, was admitted to the medical ward with a history of haematemesis. On admission to the ward he was fully conscious, orientated, pale, had cool peripheries with fresh blood around his mouth. Oxygen was commenced via mask at 35%. What would your monitoring priorities initially be?

Continued

The patient's vital signs were taken: BP 80/50, pulse 120/min and thready, respiratory rate 30/min and SpO_2 was difficult to obtain. What do these measurements tell you?

An initial diagnosis was made: hypovolaemic shock secondary to haematemesis. Intravenous access was established with two wide-bore cannulas, one in each arm. Blood was taken for LFTs, U+Es, FBC, clotting screen; cross-matched for 6 units of whole blood + 2 units of fresh frozen plasma (FFP); fluid resuscitation was commenced with Hartmann's solution. Intravenous omeprazole was administered. A urinary catheter and central venous catheter were inserted. Arterial blood gas results were within normal limits.

What monitoring would you now do?

The CVP reading is 1 mmHg. BP is now 70/50, HR 130/min, resps 30/min and the patient is becoming disorientated. Urine output is minimal and a blocked catheter is eliminated. SpO_2 is still unobtainable. What do these measurements tell you?

The patient's hypovolaemia appears to be deteriorating despite fluid resuscitation. The CVP reading is low, though caution is required as it is an isolated reading (serial readings are more helpful). The patient's conscious level continues to deteriorate, together with his vital signs. The patient required urgent transfusion and review by surgical team. Following an urgent gastroscopy, the patient was transferred to theatre for oversewing of a bleeding gastric ulcer.

CONCLUSION

Monitoring GI function is central to the management of a critically ill patient. The principles of monitoring have been discussed and include assessment of bowel action, the significance of nausea and vomiting and key aspects of monitoring for intestinal obstruction and pancreatitis.

REFERENCES

Adam, S. & Osborne, S. (2005) *Critical Care Nursing: Science and Practice* 2nd edn. Oxford Medical Publications, Oxford.

Bruce, L. & Finley, T.M.D. (1997) *Nursing in Gastroenterology.* Churchill Livingstone, London.

Felderbauer, P., Muller, C., Bulut, K. *et al.* (2005) Pathophysiology and treatment of acute pancreatitis: new therapeutic targets – a ray of hope? *Basic & Clinical Pharmacology & Toxicology* **97** (6), 342–350.

Fiore, F., Lecleire, S. & Merle, V. (2005) Changes in characteristics and outcome of acute upper gastrointestinal haemorrhage: a comparison of epidemiology and practices between 1996 and 2000 in a multicentre French study. *European Journal of Gastroenterology & Hepatology* **17** (6), 641–647.

Hawthorn, J. (1995) *Understanding and Management of Nausea and Vomiting.* Blackwell Scientific Publications, Oxford.

Herlufsen, P., Olsen, A., Carlsen, B. *et al.* (2006) Study of peristomal skin disorders in patients with permanent stomas. *British Journal of Nursing* **15** (16), 854–862.

Hollington, P., Maudsley, J., Lim, W. *et al.* (2004) An 11 year experience of enterocutaneous fistula. *British Journal of Surgery* **91** (12), 1646–1651.

Hudak, C.M., Gallo, B.M. & Morton, P.G. (1998) *Critical Care Nursing a Holistic Approach* 7th edn. Lippincott, New York.

Johnson, C. (1998) Severe acute pancreatitis: a continuing challenge for the intensive care team. *British Journal of Intensive Care* **8** (4), 130–137.

Kennedy, J. (1997) Enteral feeding for the critically ill patient. *Nursing Standard* **11** (33), 39–43.

Mallett, J. & Dougherty, L. eds. (2000) *The Royal Marsden Hospital Manual of Clinical Nursing Procedures.* Blackwell Science, Oxford.

Meadows, C. (1997) Stoma and fistula care. In: L. Bruce & T.M.D. Finley, eds *Nursing in Gastroenterology.* Churchill Livingstone, London.

Morris, A. (1992) Upper gastrointestinal haemorrhage – endoscopic approaches to diagnosis and treatment. In: I. Gilmore & R. Shields, eds. *Gastrointestinal emergencies.* W.B. Saunders, London.

Myers, A. (1998) Inside stories. *Nursing Times* **94** (20), 66–67.

Pandol, S. (2006) Acute pancreatitis. *Current Opinion in Gastroenterology* **22** (5), 481–486.

Reece-Smith, H. (1997) Pancreatitis. *Care of the Critically Ill* **13** (4), 135–138.

Renton, S., Robertson, I. & Speirs, M. (2006) Alternative management of complex wounds and fistulae. *British Journal of Nursing* **15** (16), 851–853.

Rinsema, W. (1994) *Gastrointestinal fistula: management and results of treatment.* Datawyse, Maastricht.

Robin, A., Campbell, R. & Palani, C. (1990) Total parenteral nutrition during acute pancreatitis: clinical experience with 156 patients. *World Journal of Surgery* **14**, 572–579.

Rolstad, B. & Erwin-Toth, P. (2004) Peristomal skin complications: prevention and management. *Ostomy Wound Management* **50** (9), 68–77.

Schell, H.M. & Puntillo, K.A. (2001) *Critical Care Nursing Secrets.* Hanley & Belfus, Philadelphia.

Steinberg, W. & Tenner, S. (1994) Acute pancreatitis. *New England Journal of Medicine* **330**, 1198–1210.

Talley, N.J. & O'Connor, S. (1998) *Pocket Clinical Examination*. Blackwell Science, Oxford.

Taylor, S. (1988) A guide to nasogastric feeding equipment. *Professional Nurse* **4**, 91–94.

Thompson, H.J. (1992) Post-operative nausea and vomiting. *British Journal of Theatre Nursing* **29** (5), 1130.

Winney, J. (1998) Constipation. *Nursing Standard* **13** (11), 49–56.

Woodrow, P. (2000) *Intensive Care Nursing. A Framework for Practice.* Routledge, London.

9 | Monitoring Hepatic Function

INTRODUCTION

In the context of critically ill patients, hepatic dysfunction is usually secondary to another disease process, e.g. hypoxia, hypotension (Gwinnutt 2006). Patients admitted to an ICU with a primarily non-hepatic disease frequently develop hepatic dysfunction (Hawker 1997). Acute liver failure (ALF) has a rapid progression and high mortality (Bauer *et al.* 2005; Meier *et al.* 2006). If it develops, widespread hepatocyte necrosis can lead to severely impaired hepatic function and encephalopathy. Although recovery from ALF on the ICU is usually good (Wiles 1999), overall survival is only 20–25% on medical therapy alone, with 70% requiring transplantation (Hawker 1997).

The liver, the largest organ in the body, has three broad functions: *synthesis*, *storage* and *detoxification*. Any hepatic dysfunction can affect most of the other major systems in the body. Patients with ALF frequently develop multi-organ failure and associated complications include encephalopathy, systemic infections, cerebral oedema, haemodynamic instability, coagulopathy, and renal and metabolic dysfunction (Herrera 1998). Close monitoring of hepatic function and complications of ALF is paramount; prevention or timely recognition and management of these complications is crucial (Shoemaker *et al.* 1995). Treatment is generally supportive for these patients and some ultimately will require liver transplant.

The aim of this chapter is to understand the principles of monitoring hepatic function, with specific reference to the complications of ALF.

LEARNING OBJECTIVES
At the end of the chapter the reader will be able to:

❏ outline the *functions* of the liver
❏ list the causes of *ALF*
❏ discuss the *clinical features of ALF*
❏ discuss how to monitor the specific *complications of ALF*

FUNCTIONS OF THE LIVER
The clinical features of ALF are largely attributable to the failure of normal hepatic functions (Hinds & Watson 1996). Therefore in order to appreciate the principles of monitoring hepatic function, it is essential to understand the functions of the liver, which include:

- metabolism of carbohydrates, fat, protein and bilirubin
- storage of vitamins and minerals
- detoxification of both internal and external substances
- formation and storage of glycogen
- production and storage of clotting factors prothrombin and vitamin K
- formation of amino acids and proteins, e.g. albumin
- production of heat
- manufacture and secretion of bile

(Wilson & Waugh 1996)

CAUSES OF ALF
Causes of ALF can be classified as either primary or secondary. Primary causes of ALF include:

- *paracetamol poisoning*: the commonest cause in the UK (Larrey & Pageaux, 2005)
- *drugs* (Larrey & Pageaux 2005)
- *alcohol, industrial solvents, mushrooms* (Sussman 1996)
- *hepatitis* and other viruses

  Secondary causes of ALF include:

- *hypoperfusion*, the commonest cause (Hickman & Potter 1990; Woodrow 2000)
- *sepsis*

- *fatty infiltration of the liver* precipitated by high calorie parenteral nutrition and benign post-operative cholestasis (Hinds &
  Watson 1996)
- *multiple organ failure*
  (Leach 2004; Singer & Webb 2005; Gwinnutt 2006)

CLINICAL FEATURES OF ALF

A patient with ALF will have clinical manifestations that are
directly related to the degree of impaired hepatic function
(Budden & Vink 1996). Early clinical features include nausea,
vomiting, anorexia, abdominal pain, flatulence, diarrhoea, steat-
orrhoea, pyrexia, pruritus, jaundice, loss of weight and dark urine
(Ignatavicius & Bayne 1991).

Jaundice, a yellow pigmentation of the tissues, may be observed
in the skin and conjunctiva and is a sign of abnormal bilirubin
metabolism and excretion. Although the normal serum bilirubin
is 3–13 mmol/l, jaundice may not be evident until the level has
risen to 34 mmol/l (Wilson & Waugh 1996) (other causes of jaundice include haemolysis and obstruction to the flow of bile).

Liver function tests should be performed at least daily. A
plasma bilirubin concentration of >300 mmol/l is a poor prognos-
tic sign (Hawker 1997). International normalised ratio (INR) is a
useful indicator of hepatic function.

MONITORING THE SPECIFIC COMPLICATIONS OF ALF

Encephalopathy

Encephalopathy is a characteristic clinical feature of ALF. The
exact cause is unknown, though it is possible that the accumulation of circulating toxic substances plays a key role. It is important
to recognise the early signs of encephalopathy, thus allowing
early treatment (Budden & Vink 1996). It can be classified into
four grades depending on severity (Table 9.1) and usually pro-
gresses over several days, though deep coma can develop in just
a few hours (Hinds & Watson 1996). In patients with high grades
of encephalopathy, the chances of survival are less than 20% with
medical management alone (Lai & Murphy 2004). Although it is
important to document the grade of encephalopathy, repeated

Table 9.1 Grading of hepatic encephalopathy.

Grade	Details
0	Normal mental state
1	Changes in mental state, e.g. lack of awareness, anxiety, euphoria, reduced attention span, difficulty with adding and subtracting
2	Lethargy, disorientation (for time), personality changes, inappropriate behaviour
3	Stupor, but responsive to stimuli; gross disorientation, confusion
4	Coma

Reproduced by permission of MacLennan T. Petty from 'Hepatic Encephalopathy' reproduced in Talley & O'Connor (2001) *Clinical Examination*, p. 192.

Table 9.2 Clinical examination of encephalopathy.

Grade of encephalopathy	Tone and reflexes	Response to pain	Pupils
Grade 1	Normal		
Grade 2	Brisk reflexes and increased tone	Obeys	Normal
Grade 3	Up-going plantar reflexes, clonus hippus	Localises, flexes	'Hyper-reactive'
Grade 4	Sustained clonus	Extends	Dilated, sluggish
Brain death	Flaccid, absent reflexes	None	Fixed and dilated

Reprinted from *Intensive Care Manual*, T. Oh, 4th edn, © 1997, with permission from Elsevier Inc.

clinical examination is more helpful if the clinical course is to be more accurately followed (Hawker 1997) (Table 9.2).

The neurological status of the patient should be evaluated and closely monitored; in brief, the conscious level, motor movement, sensory pupil size and reaction to light should be examined. In advanced encephalopathy the pupils may become dilated and react sluggishly to light; if they become dilated and unreactive, brainstem coning is likely (Hawker 1997).

Orientation should be monitored together with concentration span, restlessness, personality and behaviour changes, emotional lability, drowsiness, slurred or slow speech and disturbances in the sleep pattern. A generalised increase in muscle tone is an early sign of progression of encephalopathy. Spontaneous hyperventilation is common, and can result in a significant alkalosis (Hawker 1997). The respiratory rate should therefore be regularly recorded together with blood gas analysis.

Sedatives, often administered to these patients, can cause a rapid deterioration of mental status and are therefore not recommended (Shoemaker *et al*. 1995). The degree of electroencephalographic (EEG) changes correlates with the degree of cerebral dysfunction; serial EEGs together with clinical assessment can be performed to determine the patient's progress (Hinds & Watson 1996).

Cerebral oedema

Cerebral oedema is the leading cause of death in patients with ALF (Plevris *et al*. 1998; Lai & Murphy 2004), being present in over 80% of grade IV encephalopathies (Hawker 1997). The clinical signs of cerebral oedema, i.e. systemic hypertension, deceberate posturing and abnormal pupillary reflexes, are generally attributed to brainstem compression. Cerebral oedema provokes intracranial hypertension that impairs cerebral perfusion pressure.

Cerebral blood flow correlates to arterial pressure and not cardiac output in patients with ALF; strict cardiovascular control is important when pressure-passive cerebral circulation is present in order to maintain continuous and adequate cerebral oxygenation and avoid the development of cerebral hyperaemia and cerebral oedema (Larsen *et al*. 2000). Close cardiac and haemodynamic monitoring is therefore imperative.

Intracranial pressure (ICP) monitoring allows the early detection and treatment of cerebral oedema (Lockhart-Wood 1996). Although it is a well established technique, complications (Waite 1993), which are sometimes fatal (Blei *et al*. 1993), can occur. For each patient, the risk–benefit ratio should be considered, particularly as positive outcomes have been achieved without ICP monitoring (Sheil *et al*. 1991).

Coagulopathy and haemorrhaging

Patients with ALF frequently develop severe coagulopathy; the hepatic synthesis of clotting factors is impaired and as a result the clotting times, e.g. INR, partial thromboplastin time (PTT), are always prolonged. In addition qualitative and quantitative defects of platelets occur (O'Grady & Williams 1986). The prothrombin time (PT) is considered to be the most sensitive indicator of hepatic reserve in ALF (Gwinnutt 2006).

The most common site for haemorrhage is the gastrointestinal tract (Hawker 1997); other sites include the nasopharynx, respiratory tract and skin puncture sites (Hawker 1997). It is important to monitor for signs of haemorrhage, e.g. in faeces, urine, skin, sputum, endotracheal tube and vomit.

Renal failure

Renal failure is a common complication of ALF (Hinds & Watson 1996; Adam & Osborne 2005), occurring in approximately 75% of patients with grade IV encephalopathy following paracetamol overdose and in <30% of other aetiologies (O'Grady & Williams 1986). Common clinical manifestations include oliguria, increased plasma concentrations of creatinine, low sodium content in the urine and previous normal renal function (Hawker 1997). Urine output should therefore be closely monitored.

Sepsis

Bacterial infection is common, occurring in 80% of patients with ALF (Rolando *et al*. 1990; Gill & Sterling 2001). Sepsis worsens hepatic function (Rolando *et al*. 1990). Septic patients are more likely to develop renal failure and gastrointestinal haemorrhaging and have a significantly higher mortality risk than non-septic patients (Shoemaker *et al*. 1995).

The patient's vital signs should be closely monitored, though pyrexia and an increased white cell count are absent in 30% of patents with documented bacterial infection (Hawker 1997). As pulmonary and urinary tract infections are the most common (Shoemaker *et al*. 1995), sputum and urine should be scrutinised and samples sent for microbiology, culture and sensitivity.

Although ascites may be associated with ALF, spontaneous bacterial peritonitis is a rare complication (Poddar *et al*. 1998).

Metabolic disturbances

Hypoglycaemia is common, resulting from impaired gluconeo-genesis, reduced glycogen stores and increased circulating levels of insulin (Hawker 1997). Blood glucose levels should be measured regularly. Primary respiratory alkalosis is common in spontaneously breathing patients (see the section on Encephalopathy earlier). Impaired hepatic synthesis of urea and hypokalaemia can cause metabolic alkalosis. Electrolyte disturbances are very common.

Scenario

Janet, a 47-year-old woman with a history of chronic alcohol abuse, was admitted to the medical HDU with a diagnosis of hepatic failure. On admission her condition was stable with normal haemodynamic parameters. She was, however, graded at level 1 hepatic encephalopathy, due to alteration in her mood and slight confusion. She had obvious abdominal ascites, jaundice and pitting ankle oedema. Bloods were taken for analysis: LFTs, U&Es, clotting time, FBC. What are her monitoring priorities?

Her airway was monitored and she had supplementary humidified oxygen at 35%. Continuous SpO_2 monitoring and continuous ECG were instigated, along with hourly fluid balance. Regular assessment of conscious level was performed to detect any early deterioration, which is possible in these patients with encephalopathy. Blood glucose levels were monitored hourly initially, as the liver's function of gluconeogenesis is reduced and hypoglycaemia is common in such patients.

A low-protein high-carbohydrate enteral feed was commenced after ensuring that there was no active bleeding in the GI tract. Careful monitoring of the patient was performed to ascertain if active bleeding had occurred as clotting disorders are a common occurrence in liver failure due to the storage of clotting factors in the liver. After several days of careful monitoring and support, Janet's conscious state began to improve and she was transferred to the general ward for further support.

CONCLUSION

ICU patients frequently develop hepatic dysfunction. If ALF develops, widespread hepatocyte necrosis can lead to severely impaired hepatic function and life-threatening complications may result. Close monitoring of hepatic function and complications of ALF is paramount if the patient's prognosis is to improve.

REFERENCES

Adam, S. & Osborne, S. (2005) *Critical Care Nursing Science and Practice* 2nd edn. Oxford University Press, Oxford.

Bauer, M., Winning, J. & Kortgen, A. (2005) Liver failure. *Current Opinion in Anaesthesiology* **18** (2), 111–116.

Blei, A., Olafsson, S., Webster, S. & Levy, R. (1993) Complications of intracranial pressure monitoring in fulminant hepatic failure. *The Lancet* **341**, 157–158.

Budden, L. & Vink, R. (1996) Paracetamol overdose: pathophysiology and nursing management. *British Journal of Nursing* **5** (3), 145–152.

Gill, R. & Sterling, R. (2001) Acute liver failure. *Journal of Clinical Gastroenterology* **33**, 191–198.

Gwinnutt, C. (2006) *Clinical Anaesthesia* 2nd edn. Blackwell Publishing, Oxford.

Hawker, F. (1997) Hepatic failure. In: T. Oh, ed. *Intensive Care Manual* 4th edn. Butterworth Heinemann, Oxford.

Herrera, J. (1998) Management of acute liver failure. *Digestive Diseases* **16** (5), 274–283.

Hickman, P. & Potter, J. (1990) Mortality associated with ischaemic hepatitis. *Australian and New Zealand Journal of Medicine* **20**, 32–34.

Hinds, C.J. & Watson, D. (1996) *Intensive Care: a concise textbook* 2nd edn. W.B. Saunders, London.

Ignatavicius, D. & Bayne, M. (1991) *Medical-Surgical: A Nursing Process Approach*. W.B. Saunders, Philadelphia.

Lai, W. & Murphy, N. (2004) Management of acute liver failure. *Continuing Education in Anaesthesia, Critical Care and Pain* **4** (2), 40–43.

Langley, S. & Pain, J. (1994) Surgery and liver dysfunction. *Care of the Critically Ill* **10** (3), 113–117.

Larrey, D. & Pageaux, G. (2005) Drug-induced acute liver failure. *European Journal of Gastroenterology and Hepatology* **17** (2), 141–143.

Larsen, F., Strauss, G., Knudsen, G. *et al.* (2000) Cerebral perfusion, cardiac output and arterial pressure in patients with fulminant hepatic failure. *Critical Care Medicine* **28** (4), 996–1000.

Leach, R. (2004) *Critical Care Medicine at a Glance.* Blackwell Publishing, Oxford.

Lockhart-Wood, K. (1996) Developments in practice. Cerebral oedema in fulminant hepatic failure. *Nursing in Critical Care* **1** (6), 283–285.

Mallett, J. & Dougherty, L. (2000) eds. *The Royal Marsden Hospital Manual of Clinical Nursing Procedures*. Blackwell Science, Oxford.

Meier, M., Woywodt, A., Hoeper. M, *et al.* (2006) Acute liver failure: a message found under the skin. *Postgraduate Medical Journal* **81** (954), 269–270.

O'Grady, J.G. & Williams, R. (1986) Management of acute liver failure. *Schweizerische Medizidinische Wochenschrift* **116** (17), 541–544.

Oh, T. (1997) ed. *Intensive Care Manual* 4th edn. Butterworth-Heinemann, Oxford.

Plevris, J., Schina, M. & Hayes, P. (1998) Review article: the management of acute liver failure. *Alimentary Pharmacology and Therapeutics* **12** (5), 405–418.

Poddar, U., Chawla, Y., Dhiman, R. *et al.* (1998) Spontaneous bacterial peritonitis in fulminant hepatic failure. *Journal of Gastroenterology and Hepatology* **13** (1), 109–111.

Rolando, P.G., Harvey, F., Brahm, J. *et al.* (1990) Prospective study of bacterial infection in acute liver failure: an analysis of fifty patients. *Hepatology* **11**, 49–53.

Sheil, A., McCaughan, G., Isai, H. *et al.* (1991) Acute and subacute fulminant hepatic failure: the role of liver transplantation. *Medical Journal of Australia* **154**, 724–728.

Shoemaker, W., Ayres, S., Grenuik, A. & Hollrook, P. (1995) *Textbook of Critical Care*. W.B. Saunders, London.

Singer, M. & Webb, A. (2005) *Oxford Handbook of Critical Care* 2nd edn. Oxford University Press, Oxford.

Stanley, A., Lee, A. & Hayes, P. (1995) Management of acute liver failure. *British Journal of Intensive Care* **5** (1), 8–15.

Sussman, N. (1996) Fulminant hepatic failure. In: D. Zakim & T. Boyer, eds. *Hepatology: A Textbook of Liver Disease* 3rd edn. W.B. Saunders, Philadelphia.

Talley, N. & O'Connor, S. (2001) *Clinical Examination* 4th edn. MacLennan Petty, East Gardens, NSW, Australia.

Waite, L. (1993) Commentary on complications of intracranial pressure monitoring in fulminant hepatic failure. *AACN Nursing Scan in Critical Care* **3** (6), 19–20.

Wiles, C. (1999) Critical care apheresis: hepatic failure. *Therapeutic Apheresis* **3** (1), 31–33.

Wilson, K. & Waugh, A. (1996) *Anatomy and Physiology in Health and Illness* 8th edn. Churchill Livingstone, London.

Woodrow, P. (2000) *Intensive Care Nursing, A Framework for Practice*. Routledge, London.

Monitoring Endocrine Function

10

INTRODUCTION

Monitoring endocrine function is an important aspect of caring for the critically ill patient. Disorders of this function can be life threatening (Savage *et al.* 2004) and early detection of problems through close monitoring is essential.

For the purpose of this chapter, only the potentially life-threatening disorders of endocrine function will be discussed. An understanding of the physiology of the endocrine system is important if the effects of its malfunction are to be appreciated.

The aim of this chapter is to understand the principles of monitoring endocrine function.

LEARNING OBJECTIVES

At the end of the chapter the reader will be able to:

❏ discuss the principles of monitoring *pituitary gland function*
❏ outline the principles of monitoring the *endocrine function of the pancreas*
❏ discuss the principles of monitoring *adrenal gland function*
❏ outline the principles of monitoring *thyroid gland function*
❏ discuss the principles of monitoring *parathyroid gland function*

PRINCIPLES OF MONITORING PITUITARY GLAND FUNCTION

One of the functions of the pituitary gland is to secrete the antidiuretic hormone (ADH). ADH acts on the renal tubules resulting in reabsorption of water. Any damage to the posterior pituitary gland or adjacent hypothalamus, for instance following neurosurgery, head injury, malignancy or drug therapy, e.g. amiodarone, can lead to insufficient or lack of ADH secretion (Adam & Osborne 2005) which can lead to diabetes insipidus.

Diabetes insipidus

Diabetes insipidus is a syndrome that has excessive thirst, poly-dipsia and polyuria as its hallmarks (Vedig 2004a). Water loss in extreme cases can be around 20 litres per day. If untreated, diabetes insipidus can result in severe electrolyte imbalance, i.e. severe hypernatraemia and hyperosmolar states.

Monitoring priorities

Management problems on an ICU associated with diabetes insipidus are usually hypovolaemia and polyuria (Vedig 2004a). In respect of hypovolaemia, close monitoring of cardiovascular parameters is essential, including pulse, blood pressure and central venous pressure monitoring. Maintenance of strict fluid balance and daily weight is also important (Vedig 2004a).

Because patients with diabetes insipidus have an increased serum osmolarity and reduced urine osmolarity, biochemical investigations of both blood and urine are vital in the accurate monitoring of this syndrome. Specific gravity, a crude measurement, is often ignored on routine ward testing but is invaluable in this scenario: SG <1.010 is indicative of diabetes insipidus. Urine osmolarity is obtained either as a spot specimen or from a 24-hour collection. Normal values are 300–1300 mosm/kg.

Plasma osmolarity is calculated from the equation of serum sodium, potassium, glucose and urea (normal value is 275–295 mosm/kg). Regular biochemical assessment of urea and electrolytes is essential to monitor the progression of this syndrome.

PRINCIPLES OF MONITORING THE ENDOCRINE FUNCTION OF THE PANCREAS

The pancreas secretes two hormones, *insulin* and *glucagon*. Functions of insulin include lowering blood glucose levels by promoting transport of glucose into the cells, promoting glycogen storage in muscle and hepatic cells and inhibiting fat metabolism (Adam & Osborne 2005). Glucagon increases blood glucose levels.

Disturbances in pancreatic function that affect insulin production will lead to hyperglycaemia and glycosuria. If left untreated diabetic ketoacidosis will develop.

The normal fasting blood glucose level is 3.9–6.2 mmol/l (Bersten & Soni 2004). When monitoring a critically ill patient it is important to undertake regular bedside blood glucose measurements. These are particularly important if the patient is hypoglycaemic or hyperglycaemic, a known diabetic, receiving insulin or receiving nutritional support. Monitoring the patient's blood sugar can, in the short term, prevent hypoglycaemia and ketoacidosis and, in the long term, prevent disorders that affect the vascular and neural pathways (Mallett & Dougherty 2000). Blood glucose measurements are more accurate than urinalysis because the results relate to the time of testing (Cowan 1997).

Procedure for bedside blood glucose measurements

The following is adapted from the Walsall NHS Trust's procedure for 'Blood glucose estimation using the Advantage 11 machine and test strips'.

The procedure for use of the Advantage 11 meter (Fig. 10.1) is as follows

1. Wash and dry the patient's hands using soap and water. Avoid using an alcohol swab. It may contaminate the skin and lead to an inaccurate result (Burden 2001).
2. Having ensured the Advantage 11 test strips are in date, remove one from the container and insert it (yellow window facing up) into the test strip slot. The meter should turn on automatically. Replace the container top.
3. Check that the code number on the meter corresponds to the one on the test strip container. This will help ensure accuracy of the result.
4. Once the blood drop symbol flashes on the meter, prick the side of the patient's finger with a blood lancet (needles should not be used because they are designed to cut through the skin with minimal trauma resulting in insufficient blood for the test (Burden 2001)). The side of the finger is used because it is less painful for the patient and easier to obtain a hanging droplet of blood (Mallett & Dougherty 2000). As multiple 'stabbing' in the same place can increase the risk of infection, harden the

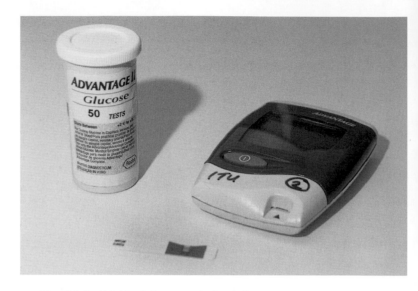

Fig. 10.1 Bedside blood glucose monitoring device.

skin and be painful for the patient the site used should be rotated (Mallett & Dougherty 2000).

5. After waiting a few seconds to allow the capillaries to relax, squeeze the patient's finger to obtain a small drop of blood, bringing it together with the test strip. The blood will be drawn automatically on to the test strip.

6. Apply a cotton wool pad or tissue to the patient's finger.

7. The test result will be displayed in mmol/l after 40 seconds. The presence of a yellow colour in the yellow window following the application of the drop of blood indicates that the test result may be erroneous. Discard the test strip and repeat the procedure.

8. Document the measurement (Fig. 10.2).

The Advantage 11 test strips should be kept in the original container, stored at room temperature (<32°C) and not refrigerated. Tests should be performed at temperatures between 14 and 40°C.

WALSALL HOSPITALS NATIONAL HEATH SERVICE TRUST

BLOOD GLUCOSE MONITORING CHART

Patients Name ....

Hospital No. .... Ward ....

DATE & TIME											
28											
24											
22											
20											
18											
16											
15											
14											
13											
12											
11											
10											
09											
08											
07											
06		This area shaded in light blue to indicate near normal range									
05											
04											
03											
02											
01											
Insulin Given											

BLOOD GLUCOSE MMOLS/L

Fig. 10.2 Blood glucose monitoring chart (Walsall Hospitals NHS Trust).

Best practice – blood glucose measurements

Use soap and water, not alcohol swab, to clean site
Ensure test strip is in date, calibrated with the machine and stored
   following manufacturer's recommendations
Do not use a needle to draw blood
Use side of patient's finger to draw blood, or preferably from an
   arterial line if in situ
Rotate finger used to avoid multiple stabbing on the same site
Allow blood to be drawn on to test strip
Ensure sufficient blood has been obtained
Be aware of factors that can affect the result
Ensure quality control procedures are carried out following local
   protocols

Blood glucose measurements may be affected by:

- *hyperosmolar hyperglycaemia*: a false low reading may be obtained (Batki *et al.* 1999)
- *hyperlipaemia* (abnormal fat concentrations): e.g. cholesterol >56.5 mmol/l
- *high levels of bilirubin* (>0.43 mmol/l, e.g. in jaundice)
- *ascorbic acid (vitamin C) infusion*
- *peritoneal dialysis*
- *haemocrit values*: if high (>55%) the blood glucose measurement may be up to 15% too low; if low (<35%) the blood glucose level may be up to 10% too high

(Medical Devices Agency 1996)

To ensure accuracy, quality control procedures using Advantage 11 glucose control solutions should be undertaken following manufacturer's recommendations. The Medical Devices Agency advises that independent quality control procedures should be regularly carried out on all extra-laboratory measurement devices (Medical Devices Agency 1996).

Newer devices are currently being developed to enable non-invasive methods of monitoring blood glucose (Burden 2001). Glucose sensors may give 24-hour blood glucose patterns, e.g. to detect unrecognised hypoglycaemia (American Diabetes Association 2001).

Hyperglycaemia and diabetic ketoacidosis

There are many causes of hyperglycaemia including diabetes mellitus, acute pancreatitis, parenteral nutrition and sepsis (Young & Oh 1997). Thirty percent of patients admitted with an acute coronary syndrome have either diabetes or stress hyperglycaemia (Savage *et al*. 2004).

Diabetic ketoacidosis results from lack of insulin (Savage *et al*. 2004). It is a serious life-threatening metabolic complication of diabetes mellitus consisting of three concurrent abnormalities: hyperglycaemia, hyperketonaemia and metabolic acidosis (Savage *et al*. 2004).

A history of infection, illness, inadequate or omitted insulin therapy is common (Kitabchi *et al*. 1983). The characteristics of diabetic ketoacidosis include hyperglycaemia, metabolic acidosis, dehydration, polyuria, glycosuria, ketonuria, weight loss, tachycardia and tachypnoea (Dunning 1994). Monitoring priorities include the following:

- *airway patency* (if the patient is semiconscious or in a coma)
- *arterial blood gas analysis*: indicated if there is altered conscious level or if breathing is compromised (Savage *et al*. 2004)
- *pulse oximetry*: breathing may be compromised
- *pulse, blood pressure and central venous pressure measurements*: hypovolaemia
- *ECG monitoring*: cardiac arrhythmias
- *blood ketones measurements*: the use of blood ketone tests is preferred to urine ketone tests for diagnosis and monitoring of diabetic ketoacidosis (American Diabetes Association 2004)
- *blood glucose measurements*: hourly (Savage *et al*. 2004) to monitor hyperglycaemia and the effect of prescribed insulin
- *strict fluid balance*: fluid replacement should be closely monitored
- *blood cultures*: to detect sepsis
- *serum potassium measurements*: to detect hypokalaemia or hyperkalaemia (Miller 1999).

Hypoglycaemia

Hypoglycaemia, which can be defined as a circulating blood glucose level of <2.0 mmol/l (Hinds & Watson 1996), usually occurs in diabetics. Causes include too much insulin or inadequate nutritional intake. It can also complicate hepatic failure, renal failure and adrenocortical insufficiency (Rossini & Mordes 1991; Vedig 2004c). Regular blood glucose measurements are required.

PRINCIPLES OF MONITORING ADRENAL GLAND FUNCTION

The adrenal glands comprise the medulla and cortex. The adrenal medulla secretes the hormones adrenaline and noradrenaline (catecholamines) in response to sympathetic stimulation. The adrenal cortex secretes three categories of hormones, all of which are steroids.

Phaeochromocytoma

Phaeochromocytoma (tumour of the adrenal medulla) can lead to the secretion of high levels of catecholamines, usually intermittently (Savage *et al.* 2004). Common symptoms include severe hypertension, headache, tachycardia, hyperglycaemia, bowel disturbances and blurred vision (Adam & Osborne 2005). Hypertension is paroxysmal initially, but later becomes sustained (Karet & Brown 1994). Monitoring priorities include:

- *arterial pressure monitoring*: hypertension
- *ECG monitoring*: cardiac arrhythmias
- *blood glucose measurements*: to monitor hyperglycaemia and evaluate treatment

Addisonian crisis

Addisonian crisis results from acute adrenocortisol insufficiency. Acute adrenocortical insufficiency can be caused by a primary failure of the adrenal gland or secondary to the lack of adrenocorticotrophic hormone (ACTH) drive from the pituitary gland (Savage *et al.* 2004). The clinical features, which relate mainly from the deficiency of aldosterone, include thirst, polyuria, dehydration, cardiac arrhythmias, electrolyte imbalance and hypotension (Adam & Osborne 2005). Monitoring priorities include:

- *arterial blood gas analysis*: metabolic and respiratory acidosis may occur

- *ECG monitoring*: cardiac arrhythmias
- *arterial pressure monitoring*: hypotension
- *central venous pressure monitoring*: hypotension
- *strict fluid balance*: polyuria
- *blood glucose measurements*: hypoglycaemia

PRINCIPLES OF MONITORING THYROID GLAND FUNCTION
The thyroid gland secretes three hormones: *thyroxine* (T3), *triiodothyronine* (T4) and *calcitonin*. T3 and T4 are responsible for the metabolic rate of all bodily tissues. Calcitonin reduces serum calcium levels. Thyroid crisis and myxoedema coma result from over- and undersecretion of the thyroid gland, respectively. If untreated they have a high mortality rate (Vedig 2004b).

Thyroid crisis
Hyperthyroidism (also known as thyrotoxicosis) results from oversecretion of T3 and T4 hormones leading to hypermetabolism. Thyroid crisis (thyroid storm) is life threatening and is the clinical extreme of hyperthyroidism (Adam & Osborne 2005).

Thyroid crisis is characterised by tachyarrhythmias, hyperpyrexia, neurological and gastrointestinal disturbances (Savage *et al.* 2004). If the patient has underlying cardiac disease or has a compromised cardiovascular system, the risk of serious complications increases. Thyroid crisis carries a relatively high mortality rate, so careful and accurate monitoring is therefore essential. Monitoring priorities include:

- respiratory rate, pulse oximetry and arterial blood gas analysis: patient may develop pulmonary oedema
- ECG monitoring: cardiac arrhythmias
- arterial blood pressure monitoring: hypotension may develop
- central venous pressure monitoring: patient can develop heart failure, there may also be considerable fluid loss
- strict fluid balance: considerable fluid loss (excessive sweating)
- blood glucose measurements: hypoglycaemia
- core temperature measurements: patient may develop extreme pyrexia (>40°C) (Adam & Osborne 2005)
- neurological monitoring: extreme agitation and coma may develop

Myxoedema coma

Myxoedema coma results from decreased T4 production and occurs most commonly in the elderly female population. There is usually a long history of hypothyroidism (Vedig 2004b). Effects include unconsciousness, hypothermia (as low as 23°C), hypoventilation, hypotension and hypoglycaemia (Savage *et al.* 2004). Monitoring priorities include:

- *airway*: unconscious patient
- *respiratory rate, pulse oximetry and arterial blood gas analysis*: hypoventilation
- *ECG monitoring*: bradycardia
- *arterial blood pressure monitoring*: hypotension
- *central venous pressure monitoring*: patient may develop heart failure, also there may be considerable fluid gain
- *strict fluid balance*: there may be considerable fluid gain
- *blood glucose measurements*: hypoglycaemia
- *core temperature measurements*: hypothermia
- *neurological monitoring*: coma

PRINCIPLES OF MONITORING PARATHYROID GLAND FUNCTION

The parathyroid glands secrete parathyroid hormone which raises serum calcium levels. Calcium is essential for a variety of bodily functions including muscle contraction, blood clotting and maintenance of cell membrane integrity. Abnormalities in parathyroid function (hyperparathyroidism and hypoparathyroidism) can lead to calcium disorders which can be life threatening.

Hypercalcaemia

Symptomatic hypercalcaemia requires urgent treatment and if it is severe the patient should be admitted to the ICU (Adam & Osborne 2005). Severe hypercalcaemia (corrected serum calcium >3.0 mmol/l) requires urgent treatment and is usually caused by malignancy (Savage *et al.* 2004). Monitoring priorities include:

- *ECG monitoring*: cardiac arrhythmias
- *arterial blood pressure monitoring*: hypertension
- *central venous pressure monitoring*: hypovolaemia
- *strict fluid balance*: dehydration, polyuria and hypovolaemia

Hypocalcaemia

Hypocalcaemia is present in approximately 70–90% of critically ill patients (Venkatesh 2004). Acute symptomatic hypocalcaemia is a medical emergency, requiring urgent treatment (Venkatesh 2004). Monitoring priorities include:

- *airway patency*
- *respirations, pulse oximetry and arterial blood gas analysis*: respiratory compromise
- *ECG monitoring*: cardiac arrhythmias
- *arterial blood pressure*: hypotension
- *central venous pressure monitoring*: hypotension
- *neurological monitoring*: convulsions and altered conscious level

---

Scenario

James, a 28-year-old man, was admitted to the HDU with a history of weight loss, general malaise, polyuria, polydipsia, lethargy and deep sighing Kussmaul respirations. He was a known diabetic but had omitted his insulin injections over the preceding few days and was also complaining of diarrhoea and vomiting. A provisional diagnosis of diabetic ketoacidosis was made. What are the monitoring priorities?

BP 90/60, pulse 125/min, respiratory rate 35/min, temp 38.5°C, SpO_2 95%, blood glucose is 40 mmol/l. The patient's vital signs were consistent with acute circulatory failure secondary to dehydration caused by excessive fluid loss. The pyrexia may be associated with the diarrhoea and vomiting. Blood glucose measurements and urinalysis were undertaken. The presence of hyperglycaemia, glycosuria, ketonuria and ketonaemia helped to confirm the diagnosis of diabetic ketoacidosis.

Arterial blood gas results are as follows:

pH 7.1
$PaCO_2$ 2.9 kPa (15 mmHg)
PaO_2 11.8 kPa (88.5 mmHg)
HCO_3^- 12 mmol/l
BE −13
SaO_2 97%

What do the arterial blood gases show?

Continued

> *The patient has metabolic acidosis with respiratory compensation. He is hyperventilating in order to excrete more carbon dioxide, therefore reducing the level of free hydrogen ions available.*
>
> Strict fluid balance monitoring was initiated. Aggressive intravenous fluid replacement was also commenced together with an insulin infusion to treat the hyperglycaemia. ECG monitoring was essential as hypokalaemia (potassium <2.8 mmol/l) was present. Intravenous potassium therapy was also commenced. Ongoing monitoring priorities include vital signs, arterial blood gases, ECG monitoring, blood glucose measurements, urinalysis, fluid balance and any vomiting/bowel action. In addition it is important to monitor the patient's conscious level as unconsciousness may ensue.

CONCLUSION

Monitoring endocrine function is an important aspect of caring for the critically ill patient. Brief details on normal physiology, in relation to each endocrine gland function, have been provided. The priorities of monitoring endocrine function have been highlighted.

REFERENCES

Adam, S. & Osborne, S. (2005) *Critical Care Nursing: Science and Practice* 2nd edn. Oxford Medical Publications, Oxford.

American Diabetes Association (2001) Clinical practice recommendations. *Diabetes Care* **24**, (Supplement) S80–S82.

American Diabetes Association (2004) Clinical practice recommendations 2004. *Diabetes Care* **27**, (Supplement 1) S94–S102.

Batki, A.., Holder, R., Thomason, H. *et al.* (1999) Selecting blood glucose monitoring systems. *Professional Nurse* **14** (10), 715–723.

Bersten, A. & Soni, N. (2004) eds. *Intensive Care Manual* 5th edn. Butterworth Heinemann, Oxford.

Burden, M. (2001) Diabetes: blood glucose monitoring. *Nursing Times* **97** (8), 37–39.

Cowan, T. (1997) Blood glucose monitoring devices. *Professional Nurse* **12** (8), 593–597.

Dunning, T. (1994) *Care of People with Diabetes*. Blackwell Science, Oxford.

Hinds, C.J. & Watson, D. (1996) *Intensive Care: A Concise Textbook* 2nd edn. W.B. Saunders, London.

Karet, F. & Brown, M. (1994) Phaeochromocytoma: diagnosis and management. *Postgraduate Medical Journal* **70**, 326–328.

Kitabchi, A., Fisher, J., Matteri, R. & Murphy, M. (1983) The use of continuous insulin delivery systems in the treatment of diabetes mellitus. *Advances in International Medicine* **28**, 449–490.

Mallett, J. & Dougherty, L. (2000) eds *The Royal Marsden Hospital Manual of Clinical Nursing Procedures*. Blackwell Science, Oxford.

Medical Devices Agency Adverse Incident Centre (1996) Safety Notice 9616: *Extra-laboratory use of blood glucose meters and test strips: contra-indications, training and advice to users*. Medical Devices Agency, London.

Miller, J. (1999) Management of diabetic ketoacidosis. *Journal of Emergency Nursing* **25** (6), 514–519.

Oh, T. (1997) ed. *Intensive Care Manual* 4th edn. Butterworth Heinemann, Oxford.

Rossini, Λ. & Mordes, J. (1991) The diabetic comas. In: J. Rippe, R. Irwin., J. Albert & M. Fink eds, *Intensive Care Medicine.* Little Brown, Boston.

Savage, M., Mah, P., Weetman, A. & Newell-Price, J. (2004) Endocrine emergencies. *Postgraduate Medical Journal* **80**, 506–551.

Scheinkestel, C. & Oh, T. (1997) Acute calcium disorders. In: T. Oh, ed. *Intensive Care Manual* 4th edn. Butterworth Heinemann, Oxford.

Vedig, A. (2004a) Diabetes insipidus. In: A. Bersten & N. Soni eds. *Intensive Care Manual* 5th edn. Butterworth Heinemann, Oxford.

Vedig, A. (2004b) Adrenocortical insufficiency. In: A. Bersten & N. Soni eds. *Intensive Care Manual* 5th edn. Butterworth Heinemann, Oxford.

Vedig, A. (2004c) Thyroid emergencies. In: A. Bersten & N. Soni eds. *Intensive Care Manual* 5th edn. Butterworth Heinemann, Oxford.

Venkatesh, B. (2004) Acute calcium disorders. In: A. Bersten & N. Soni eds. *Intensive Care Manual* 5th edn. Butterworth Heinemann, Oxford.

Watkins, P. (1998) *ABC of Diabetes* 4th edn. BMJ Publishing Group, London.

Young, K. & Oh, T. (1997) Diabetic emergencies. In: T. Oh, ed. *Intensive Care Manual* 4th edn. Butterworth Heinemann, Oxford.

11 Monitoring Nutritional Status

INTRODUCTION

A survey carried out by McWhirter and Pennington (1994) found that 40% of patients were malnourished during their stay in hospital. Both medical and nursing staff often fail to assess and monitor nutritional status (Lennard-Jones *et al*. 1995), particularly in ICU patients (Adam 1994; Briggs 1996). Malnutrition is prevalent in many ventilated patients and its incidence on the ICU could be as high as 50% (McCain 1993).

Malnutrition leads to poor wound healing, complications post surgery and sepsis (Singer & Webb 2005). Malnourished patients have poorer outcomes following medical treatment or surgery (Kennedy 1997; Say 1997), particularly those with a weight loss greater than 10%. Early nutritional support, together with ongoing monitoring of nutritional status, should be considered in all critically ill patients (Singer & Webb 2005; Doig & Simpson 2006). A nutritional support feeding algorithm improves the nutritional support of intensive care patients and leads to greater consistency in nursing practices with respect to aspiration of gastric content and monitoring the delivery of nutrients to critically ill patients (Woien & Bjork 2006).

The aim of this chapter is to understand the principles of monitoring nutritional status.

LEARNING OBJECTIVES

At the end of the chapter the reader will be able to:

❏ discuss the *importance* of assessing nutritional status
❏ outline *how to assess* nutritional status
❏ list the factors that can *affect* nutritional status
❏ discuss the principles of monitoring *enteral feeding*
❏ discuss the principles of monitoring *total parenteral nutrition*

IMPORTANCE OF ASSESSING NUTRITIONAL STATUS

All critically ill patients have either a serious illness, have suffered major trauma and/or have had major surgery; the stress response to trauma and/or injury results in a hypermetabolic state and increased nutritional demands (Verity 1996). Severe protein-calorie malnutrition is the main problem in many ICU patients because of the high catabolic rate associated with acute critical illness and the common presence of previous chronic wasting conditions (Webb *et al*. 1999).

The effects of absent nutritional intake in critically ill patients include mucosal atrophy, loss of body tissue, skeletal muscle atrophy and weakness, immunosuppression and delayed wound healing (Verity 1996; Singer & Webb 2005); these effects may occur within days (Farquhar 1993). In particular it is now recognised that maintaining gut integrity is important to help prevent sepsis and to support the immune defence system (Albarran & Price 1998). Over-feeding can lead to hyperglycaemia and fatty infiltration of the liver (Singer & Webb 2005).

ASSESSMENT OF THE PATIENT'S NUTRITIONAL STATUS

Bedside nutritional assessment should identify patients already suffering from malnutrition and those at risk of malnutrition; early referral for nutritional support together with ongoing monitoring is essential.

Objectives of assessment

The objectives of this assessment are to:

- determine the existing *nutritional status* of the patient
- identify if the patient is *malnourished*
- provide a baseline for *monitoring* nutritional status
- ascertain the patient's *nutritional requirements*

Assessment

There is no gold standard for determining the nutritional status of patients (Arrowsmith 1999). However as any one single method can have shortcomings, it it recommended to use two or three methods in parallel to overcome this problem (McLaren & Green 1998; Quirk 2000). The different methods of nutritional assessment in patients requiring intensive care will now be discussed.

A 24-hour recall of dietary intake, food diaries and taking a dietary history are all frequently used in clinical practice (Arrowsmith 1999). A diet history can provide information on food frequency, food preferences, food allergies, portion sizes and changes in food intake.

A clinical examination can help to determine whether nutrition is inadequate (Dobb 1997) and recommended simple measurements include:

- height
- weight
- mid-upper-arm circumferences (low = overall weight loss)
- triceps skinfold thickness (low = significant depletion of fat stores)
- mid-arm muscle circumference (low = protein depletion)

(Woodrow 2000)

Regular measurements of skinfold thickness can provide an indication of oedema or dehydration and whether fat is being used as an energy source. However, in the critically ill patient this measurement may be unreliable (Taylor & Goodinson-McLaren 1992; Adam & Osborne 2005).

The patient's body mass index (BMI) can be used to calculate the nutritional status of the patient (Albarran & Price 1998). This is determined by the patient's weight and height. Nomograms are available that can aid calculation. Unfortunately regular BMI estimations are difficult in critically ill patients (Endacott 1993).

The measurement of serum albumin levels is not a good indicator of nutritional status (Horwood 1990), because a fall is more likely to result from albumin's metabolism, reflecting the severity and duration of stress, rather than nutritional status (Quirk 2000).

Muscle atrophy may be masked by gross oedema and deceptive increases in body weight (Say 1997) and can also result from prolonged immobility. Urinalysis (presence of ketones) and blood glucose monitoring are helpful.

Metabolic monitoring using indirect calorimetry can be very helpful (Adam & Osborne 2005). At present, it is the only clinical method that can provide an accurate assessment of a patient's

Table 11.1 The Harris–Benedict equation for calculating basal metabolic rate.

Men	Energy expenditure = 66.5 + (13.7 × weight in kg) + (5 × height in cm) − (6.78 × age in years)
Women	Energy expenditure = 66.5 + (9.56 × weight in kg) + (1.85 × height in cm) − (4.68 × age in years)
Injury factors	Minor operation × 1.2 Trauma × 1.3 Sepsis × 1.6 Severe burns × 2.1

energy requirements (McClave *et al.* 2001). An open-circuit metabolic monitor, attached to the ventilator, can sample inspiratory and expiratory oxygen and carbon dioxide and can provide a continuous measurement of energy expenditure (Adam 1994). However, it is inaccurate if the patient is receiving oxygen concentrations of 60% or more (Albarran & Price 1998).

There are several empirical formulae and nomograms that can be used to calculate the basal metabolic rate, the Harris–Benedict (1919) equation (Table 11.1) being the most well known (Quirk 2000). However in critically ill patients, baseline calculation errors can occur because the ideal weight and height are rarely known (Quirk 2000).

FACTORS THAT CAN AFFECT NUTRITIONAL STATUS

Common factors that can affect nutritional status in critically ill patients include:

- inability to take oral diet
- diarrhoea
- glucose intolerance
- renal dysfunction
- pain
- nausea/vomiting
- physical disability
- restricted fluid intake
- delayed gastric emptying
- fasting prior to procedures/investigations

PRINCIPLES OF MONITORING ENTERAL FEEDING

If the patient is able to take diet and fluids orally, it is important to monitor intake closely to ensure that hydration and nutritional needs are being met. Sip-feed supplements, e.g. Complan, Build Up, may improve clinical outcome (Larsson *et al*. 1990) and food charts are useful as long as they are accurately completed.

If food and sip feeding fails to meet nutritional requirements or if the patient is unable to tolerate oral diet, enteral feeding should be considered. Enteral feeding, defined as the administration of nutrients via the gastrointestinal tract (Bruce & Finley 1997), is preferable if it can be given without risk (Wernerman 2005); sometimes optimal nutritional support may necessitate the concomitant administration of enteral nutrition together with total parenteral nutrition (Woodcock & MacFie 2004).

Benefits of enteral feeding

Benefits of enteral feeding include:

- improved function of the gut and liver
- reduced incidence of stress ulceration and GI bleeding (Leach 2004)
- enhanced immune function, reduced infection rates and lower sepsis rates compared to parenteral feeding (Moore *et al*. 1992; Leary *et al*. 2000)
- possible prevention of bacterial translocation (passage of bacteria or endotoxins across the intestinal epithelium to the portal venous lymphatics, which may lead to sepsis) (Botterill & MacFie 2000)
- improved survival rates in critically ill patients (Methany 1996)
- promotion of wound healing (Heyland 1998)

Routes of enteral feeding

Routes of enteral feeding:

- *nasogastric*: tube through the nose into the stomach
- *nasoenteric*: tube through the nose into the jejunum or duodenum
- *gastrostomy or jejunostomy*: tube surgically or percutaneously inserted into the stomach or jejunum

(Singer & Webb 2005)

Nasogastric feeding
Nasogastric feeding is often started through a wide-bore (12–14 FG) tube. This allows aspiration of gastric contents to confirm tube placement and feed tolerance and facilitates the administration of medications. Wide-bore tubes are less likely to occlude than fine-bore tubes, but their long-term use is not recommended. Following insertion of a wide-bore tube, which should be radio-opaque so that the tip can be visualised on a chest radiograph, it is important to ensure correct tube placement by observing the following precautions:

- Auscultating over the stomach following injection of air via the tube: this method may only be 60% reliable (Methany *et al.* 1990).
- Aspirating gastric contents and testing the pH; if the naso-gastric tube is in the stomach and in contact with acidic gastric contents the aspirate will turn blue litmus paper red. N.B. The result may be affected if the patient is taking H_2 agonists or if the nasogastric tube is in the duodenum (Adam 1994).

Continuous enteral feeding reduces gastric acidity and increases the risk of pneumonia (Jacobs *et al.* 1990; Lee *et al.* 1990). Rest periods are therefore recommended, usually of at least 4 hours (Goldhill 2000), though at present there is no evidence determining the optimum length of time (Woodrow 2000).

Aspiration of gastric contents should be undertaken every 4–6 hours to assess gastric residual volume and provide an indication to feed tolerance. This is particularly important in the initial period when enteral feeding is being established (Raper & Maynard 1992). If the patient vomits it is usual practice to continue the feed at 10 ml/hour.

In addition aspiration is usually undertaken 1 hour following the interruption of feeding, by which time gastric emptying should have occurred (Woodrow 2000). Discarding aspirated volumes may cause an electrolyte imbalance (Methany 1993). It is therefore recommended to return all aspirates of <200 ml via the nasogastric tube (Goldhill 2000). Patients who are ventilated may have normal gastric emptying despite the lack of bowel sounds (Shelly & Church 1987). Opiates and increased intracranial pressure can impair gastric emptying (Norton *et al.* 1988).

Complications associated with wide-bore tubes include the following:

- *Nasal/oesophageal ulceration and airway/gastrointestinal haemorrhage*: more prevalent than with fine-bore tubes (Bettany & Powell-Tuck 1997).
- *Transbronchial insertion*: misplacement rates vary between 0.9% (Methany *et al.* 1990) and 2.4% (Payne-James 1988).
- *Sinusitis.*
- *Regurgitation and aspiration of gastric contents*: particularly in unconscious and ventilated patients. The presence of a nasogastric tube renders the gastro-oesophageal sphincter incompetent allowing reflux of gastric contents; a cuffed endotracheal tube does not guarantee 100% protection from aspiration (Hinds & Watson 1996). The nurse should be alert to the possibility of aspiration and should monitor the patient's respiratory function together with the consistency of suction contents.
- *Tube migration*: the tube should be well secured and marked to facilitate the early detection of migration; it should also be regularly monitored (Methany 1993). The blue litmus test on aspirated gastric contents should be undertaken regularly.
- *Risk of nosocomial pneumonia*: wide-bore tubes facilitate the migration of gut commensals into the respiratory tract particularly in the presence of H_2 blockers.
- *Tube blockage.*

Nasoenteric feeding

Nasoenteric feeding requires the use of fine-bore tubes, which are better tolerated by patients, can remain *in situ* for longer periods and cause less mucosal erosion and irritation (Raper & Maynard 1992). The feed is usually continuous and administered at a slower rate because the small intestine is unable to tolerate sudden rate changes or bolus feedings (Grodner *et al.* 1996).

Correct tube placement must be confirmed by radiography (Moxham & Goldstone 1994). Unfortunately fine-bore tubes can collapse following the application of negative pressure by a syringe, thus making them more difficult to aspirate. This may lead to decreased nursing vigilance in assessing gastric contents (Sands 1991).

Complications associated with fine-bore tubes include the following:

- *misplacement*: 0.3–4.0% of insertions (Dobb 1997)
- *tube migration* (Biggart *et al.* 1987): coughing and vomiting can dislodge the tube, increasing the risk of aspiration (Kennedy 1997). Check the gastric pH if high reflux is present or if H_2 antagonists are being used
- *guide-wire induced trauma*: e.g. oesophageal, gastric and abdominal perforation and a pneumothorax
- *tube blockage*

As the tube is placed past the pylorus (gastric–duodenal sphincter), the risk of regurgitation and aspiration of gastric contents is reduced (Hudak *et al.* 1998).

Complications of enteral feeding

Complications of enteral feeding are more commonly associated with patients requiring intensive care (Dobb 1990). The most significant ones are listed below:

- *Regurgitation and aspiration of gastric contents*: this is more common in the unconscious patient, supine patient (Ibanez *et al.* 1992) and older patient (Mullen *et al.* 1992). The presence of a wide-bore tube renders the gastro-oesophageal sphincter incompetent (Hinds & Watson 1996). Nurses need to observe suction. If possible, the patient's 'head end' should be maintained at 45 degrees.
- *Tube obstruction*: if the feed is stopped, the tube should be flushed with 10–20 ml of sterile water; if the tube is not in use it should be capped off after flushing in order to trap a column of water in the tube (Taylor 1988).
- *Diarrhoea*: associated with hyperosmolar feed and antibiotic usage.
- *Abdominal distension*: if there is poor gastric emptying or rapid infusion of feed. This is also an indication of failure to absorb

the feed; careful monitoring is essential in order to prevent perforation of the intestines (Raper & Maynard 1992).
- *Hyperglycaemia.*
- *Mild hepatic dysfunction.*

Best practice – nasogastric feeding

Use fine-bore tube whenever possible
Always confirm tube position before commencement of feed
Monitor tube position during feeding
Monitor the patient's vital signs, particularly airway
Administer feed following local guidelines, ensuring breaks as
    appropriate
Ensure feed is in date and administered following manufacturer's
    recommendations
Monitor absorption of feed
Always use clean syringe and receptacle when aspirating
Maintain fluid balance
Monitor bowel function
Monitor patient's blood chemistry

Percutaneous jejunostomy and percutaneous endoscopic gastrostomy (PEG)

PEG is the preferred method for long-term access to the GI tract (Pollard 2000). Complications include leaks, wound infection and peritonitis (Adams *et al.* 1986). The insertion site should be closely monitored, particularly as gastric contents can leak around it leading to excoriation, skin breakdown and possible wound dehiscence (Kennedy 1997). Misplacement of the tube can occur leading to peritonitis.

PRINCIPLES OF MONITORING TOTAL PARENTERAL NUTRITION

Total parenteral nutrition (TPN) (Fig. 11.1) involves the intravenous infusion of nutrients. It can be administered either peripherally or centrally, but has not been shown to reduce mortality (Heyland 1998). It should only be considered when the GI tract is not functioning. Indications include:

- ileus
- acute pancreatitis
- inflammatory bowel disease
- short bowel syndrome
- malabsorption syndromes
- multiple organ failure
- post oesophagectomy
- severe catabolic states, e.g. extensive burns, sepsis and trauma

(Gwinnutt 2006)

Table 11.2 provides a comprehensive guide to the relevant monitoring required when a patient is receiving TPN. In particular the nurse should be alert to the possible complications of TPN, which can cause death in 0.2% of patients (Wolfe *et al.* 1986).

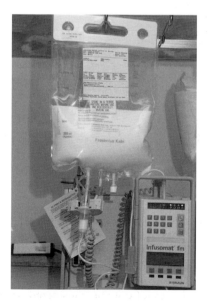

Fig. 11.1 Parenteral nutrition.

Table 11.2 Parenteral nutrition – relevant monitoring.

Monitoring	Specific tasks
Regular clinical	Nursing observations
	Temperature
	Blood pressure
	Pulse rate
	Respiratory rate
	Fluid balance
Regular ward testing	Medical assessment
	Urinalysis
	Dextrostix
	Reflectance meter
	Blood glucose
Daily (at least)	Fluid balance review
	Nutrient input review
	Biochemistry
	Serum electrolytes
	Serum urea/creatinine
	Blood glucose
Weekly (at least)	Complete blood count
	Coagulation screen
	Weight
	Liver functions tests
	Serum calcium/magnesium/phosphate
As indicated	Serum lipids
	Urine zinc
	Serum uric acid
	Blood gases
	24-hour urinary urea, electrolytes, osmolality
Special circumstances	Nitrogen balance
	Body composition
	Body protein turnover
	Gas exchange measurements
	Trace element balance
	Vitamin assays

Reproduced by permission of Butterworth-Heinemann from Oh 1997.

During TPN administration, there is a significant risk of morbidity through catheter-related sepsis and also metabolic and mechanical problems (Heenan 1996). Infection is the biggest problem (Phillips 1997), with infection rates for TPN catheters as high as 6%, compared to 1.5% for jejunostomy tubes (Schears & Deutschman 1997). Careful aseptic techniques are paramount (McGee *et al.* 1993); the entire infusion line should be dedicated to TPN use, unnecessary manipulation of the line and use of three-way stopcocks is not recommended (Phillips 1997).

Hyperosmolar dehydration syndrome can complicate hyperglycaemia; urine levels of glucose of >2% and a sudden rise in urine volumes are clinical features of osmotic diuresis (Phillips 1997). In addition, rebound hypoglycaemia can occur if the TPN infusions are abruptly stopped. Regular urinalysis and blood glucose monitoring are therefore important.

The function of the gut should be monitored so that conversion to enteral nutrition can be initiated as soon as possible. TPN should be gradually withdrawn in order to avoid complications, e.g. rebound hypoglycaemia (Phillips 1997). If TPN is delivered intermittently the catheter should be flushed with heparinised normal saline in order to minimise the risk of clot formation (Cottee 1995).

Best practice – parenteral feeding

Only use when enteral route is not possible
Do not use feed bag if there are signs of contamination
Administer feed following local protocols
Ensure entire infusion line is dedicated to parenteral nutrition use
Ensure feed and tubing are regularly changed
Monitor patient's blood chemistry
Monitor patient for complications of parenteral nutrition, particularly
    infection
Regularly flush line when not in use to maintain patency
Monitor gut function so that enteral feeding can be commenced as
    soon as possible

Scenario

Mr Brown was admitted to the ICU with an atypical pneumonia. He was sedated and ventilated with midazolam and morphine. A fine-bore nasogastric tube was inserted and the position verified by the litmus paper test and radiography. Enteral feeding was then commenced (standard feed) at 30 ml/hour. After 4 hours 100 ml is aspirated. What would you do?

As the aspirate is <200 ml, it is replaced because of its constituents:

• gastric acid reduces the proliferation of bacteria
• gastrin promotes the growth and repair of the gastric mucosa
• intrinsic factor facilitates the absorption of vitamin B12 from the gut

The enteral feed was increased to 60 ml/hour. After 4 hours 300 ml was aspirated. What would you do?

200 ml was replaced while 100 ml was discarded and the feed reduced to 30 ml/hour. After 4 hours 400 ml was aspirated. Again 200 ml was replaced and the rest discarded. The enteral feed was then re-started at 30 ml/hour. Shortly after recommencement of the feed, the patient vomited. What would you do?

Nil was aspirated and the feed was reduced to 10 ml/hour continuously and the prokinetic drug metoclopramide 10 mg IV prescribed three times daily. The following day the feed was gradually increased following the above process until a desired rate of 90 ml/hour was reached. Eight-hourly monitoring of aspirate, urea and electrolytes, fluid balance and bowel movements ensured a successful enteral feeding regime.

CONCLUSION

Nutritional status should be assessed and monitored in all critically ill patients. The method of nutritional support should also be closely monitored, in particular the patient's tolerance of it. The nurse should also be alert to possible complications.

REFERENCES

Adam, S. (1994) Aspects of current research in enteral nutrition in the critically ill. *Care of the Critically Ill* **10** (6), 246–251.
Adam, S. & Osborne, S. (2005) *Critical Care Nursing: Science and Practice* 2nd edn. Oxford University Press, Oxford.

Adams, M., Seabrook, G., Quebbeman, E. & Condon, R. (1986) Jejunostomy: a rarely indicated procedure. *Annals of Surgery* **121**, 236–238.

Albarran, J. & Price, T. (1998) *Managing the Nursing Priorities in Intensive Care*. Quay Books/Mark Allen Publishing, Dinton.

Allison, S. (1984) Nutritional problems in intensive care. *Hospital Update* **10** (12), 1001–1012.

Arrowsmith, H. (1999) A critical evaluation of the use of nutritional screening tools by nurses. *British Journal of Nursing* **8** (22), 1483–1490.

Bettany, G. & Powell-Tuck, J. (1997) Nutritional support in surgery. *Surgery* **15** (10), 233–237.

Biggart, M., McQuillan, P., Choudhry, A. & Nickalls, R. (1987) Dangers of placement of narrow-bore nasogastric feeding tubes. *Annals of the Royal College of Surgeons of England* **69**, 119–121.

Botterill, I. & MacFie, J. (2000) Bacterial translocation in the critically ill: a review of the evidence. *Care of the Critically Ill* **16** (1), 6–11.

Briggs, D. (1996) Nasogastric feeding in intensive care units: a study. *Nursing Standard* **49** (10), 42–45.

Bruce, L. & Finley, T.M.D. (1997) *Nursing in Gastroenterology*. Churchill Livingstone, London.

Cottee, S. (1995) Heparin lock practice in total parenteral nutrition. *Professional Nurse* **11** (1), 25–29.

Dobb, G. (1990) Enteral nutrition. *Clinical Anaesthesiology* **4**, 531–557.

Dobb, G. (1992) Enteral nutrition for the critically ill. In: J. Vincent, ed. *Yearbook of Intensive Care and Emergency Medicine*. Springer Verlag, Berlin.

Dobb, G. (1997) Enteral nutrition. In: T. Oh, ed. *Intensive Care Manual*, 4th edn. Butterworth Heinemann, Oxford.

Doig, G. & Simpson, F. (2006) Early enteral nutrition in the critically ill: do we need more evidence or better evidence? *Current Opinion in Critical Care* **12** (2), 126–130.

Endacott, R. (1993) Nutritional support for critically ill patients. *Nursing Standard* **7** (52), 25–28.

Farquhar, I. (1993) Parenteral nutrition in the critically ill. *Current Anaesthesia and Critical Care* **4**, 95–102.

Goldhill, D. (2000) Feeding critically ill patients. *Care of the Critically Ill* **16** (1), 20–21.

Grodner, M., Long Anderson, S., de Young, S. *et al.* (1996) *Foundations and Clinical Applications of Nutrition: A Nursing Approach*. Mosby Yearbook, St Louis MO.

Gwinnutt, C. (2006) *Clinical Anaesthesia* 2nd edn. Blackwell Publishing, Oxford.

Hamilton, H. (2000) *Total Parenteral Nutrition*. Churchill Livingstone, London.

Harris, J. & Benedict, F. (1919) *A Biometric Study of Basal Metabolism in Man*. Carnegie Institute, Washington DC.

Heenan, A. (1996) Fluids used in total parenteral nutrition. *Professional Nurse* **7**, 467–470.

Heyland, D. (1998) Nutritional support in the critically ill patient. *Critical Care Clinics* **14** (3), 423–440.

Hinds, C.J. & Watson, D. (1996) *Intensive Care: A Concise Textbook*, 2nd edn. W.B. Saunders, London.

Horwood, A. (1990) Malnourishment in intensive care units as high as 50%: are nurses doing enough to change this? *Intensive Care Nursing* **8** (3), 185–188.

Hudak, C.M., Gallo, B.M. & Morton, P.G. (1998) *Critical Care Nursing a holistic approach*, 7th edn. Lippincott, New York.

Ibanez, J., Penafiel, A., Raurich, J. *et al.* (1992) Gastroesophageal reflux (GER) in intubated patients receiving enteral nutrition: effect of supine and semirecumbent positions. *Journal of Parenteral and Enteral Nutrition* **16**, 419–422.

Jacobs, S., Chang, R., Lee, B. *et al.* (1990) Continuous enteral feeding: a major cause of pneumonia among ventilated patients. *Journal of Parenteral and Enteral Nutrition* **14**, 353–356.

Kennedy, J. (1997) Enteral feeding for the critically ill patient. *Nursing Standard* **11** (33), 39–43.

Larca, L. & Greenbaum, D. (1982) Effectiveness of intensive nutritional regimes in patients who fail to wean from mechanical ventilation. *Critical Care Medicine* **10**, 297–300.

Larsson, J., Knossan, M., Er, A. *et al.* (1990) Effect of dietary supplement on nutritional status and clinical outcome in 501 geriatric patients: a randomised study. *Clinical Nutrition* **9** (4), 179–184.

Leach, R. (2004) *Critical Care Medicine at a Glance.* Blackwell Publishing, Oxford.

Leary, T., Fellows, I. & Fletcher, S. (2000) Enteral nutrition. *Care of the Critically Ill* **16** (1), 22–27.

Lee, B., Chang, R. & Jacobs, S. (1990) Intermittent nasogastric feeding: a simple and effective method to reduce pneumonia among ventilated ICU patients. *Clinical Intensive Care* **1** (3), 100–102.

Lennard-Jones, J., Arrowsmith, H., Davison, C. *et al.* (1995) Screening by nurses and junior doctors to detect malnutrition when patients are first assessed in hospital. *Clinical Nutrition* **14**, 336–340.

Levinson, M. & Bryce, A. (1993) Enteral feeding, gastric colonisation and diarrhoea in critically ill patients: is there a relationship? *Anaesthesia and Intensive Care* **21** (1), 85–88.

Mallett, J. & Dougherty, L. (2000) eds *The Royal Marsden Hospital Manual of Clinical Nursing Procedures* 5th edn. Blackwell Science, Oxford.

McCain, R. (1993) A sensible approach to the nutritional support of mechanically ventilated critically ill patients. *Intensive Care Medicine* **19**, 129–139.

McClave, S., Snider, H., Lowen, C. *et al.* (1992) Use of residual volume as a marker for enteral feeding intolerance: prospective blinded comparison with physical examination and radiographic findings. *Journal of Parenteral and Enteral Nutrition* **16**, 419–422.

McClave, S., McClain, C. & Snider, H. (2001) Should indirect calorimetry be used as part of nutritional assessment? *Journal of Clinical Gastroenterology* **33**, 14–19.

McGee, W., Ackerman, B., Rouben, L. *et al.* (1993) Accurate placement of central venous catheters: a prospective, randomised, multicenter trial. *Critical Care Medicine* **21**, 1118–1123.

McLaren, S. & Green, S. (1998) Nutritional screening and assessment. *Professional Nurse* **13** (6), Study Supplement, S9–S14.

McWhirter, J. & Pennington, C. (1994) Incidence and recognition of malnutrition in hospital. *British Medical Journal* **308**, 945–948.

Methany, N. (1993) Minimising respiratory complications of nasogastric tube feedings: state of the science. *Heart and Lung* **22** (3), 213–222.

Methany, N. (1996) *Fluid and Electrolyte Balance: Nursing Considerations*, 3rd edn. Lippincott, Philadelphia.

Methany, N., Dettenmeier, P., Hampton, K. *et al.* (1990) Detection of inadvertent respiratory placement of small-bore feeding tubes: a report of 10 cases. *Heart and Lung* **19**, 631–638.

Moore, F., Feliciano, D., Andrassy, R. *et al.* (1992) Early enteral feeding, compared with parenteral, reduces postoperative septic complications. *Annals of Surgery* **216** (2), 172–183.

Moxham, J. & Goldstone, J. (1994) *Assisted Ventilation* 3rd edn. BMJ Publishing, London.

Mullen, H., Roubenoff, R.A. & Roubenoff, A. (1992) Risk of pulmonary aspiration among patients receiving enteral nutritional support. *Journal of Parenteral and Enteral Nutrition* **16**, 160–164.

Norton, J., Ott, L., McClain, C. *et al.* (1988) Intolerance to enteral feeding in the brain injured patient. *Journal of Neurosurgery* **68**, 62–66.

Oh, T. (1997) ed. *Intensive Care Manual* 4th edn. Butterworth-Heinemann, Oxford.

Payne-James, J. (1988) Enteral nutrition: clinical applications. *Intensive Therapy and Clinical Monitoring* **7**, 239–246.

Phillips, G. (1997) Parenteral nutrition. In: T. Oh ed., *Intensive Care Manual* 4th edn. Butterworth-Heinemann, Oxford.

Pollard, C. (2000) A PEG service with nurses at its heart. *Nursing Times* **96** (39), 39–40.

Quirk, J. (2000) Malnutrition in critically ill patients in intensive care units. *British Journal of Nursing* **9** (9), 537–541.

Raper, S. & Maynard, N. (1992) Feeding the critically ill patient. *British Journal of Nursing* **1** (6), 273–280.

Sands, J. (1991) Incidence of pulmonary aspiration in intubated patients receiving enteral nutrition through wide- and narrow-bore nasogastric feeding tubes. *Heart Lung* **20**, 75–80.

Say, J. (1997) Nutritional assessment in clinical practice: a review. *Nursing in Critical Care* **2** (1), 29–33.

Schears, G. & Deutschman, C. (1997) Common nutritional issues in paediatric and adult critical care medicine. *Critical Care Clinics* **13** (3), 669–690.

Shelly, M. & Church, J. (1987) Bowel sounds during intermittent positive pressure ventilation. *Anaesthesia* **42**, 207–209.

Singer, M. & Webb, A. (2005) *Oxford Handbook of Critical Care* 2nd edn. Oxford University Press, Oxford.

Solomon, S. & Kirby, D. (1990) The refeeding syndrome: a review. *Journal of Parenteral and Enteral Nutrition* **14**, 90–97.

Taylor, S. (1988) A guide to nasogastric feeding equipment. *Professional Nurse* **4**, 91–94.

Taylor, S. & Goodinson-McLaren, S. (1992) *Nutritional Support: A Team Approach*. Wolfe Publishing, London.

Verity, S. (1996) Nutrition and its importance to intensive care patients. *Intensive and Critical Care Nursing* **12**, 71–78.

Webb, A., Shapiro, M., Singer, M. & Surter, P. (1999) *The Oxford Textbook of Critical Care*. Oxford Medical, Oxford.

Wernerman, J. (2005) Guidelines for nutritional support in intensive care unit patients: a critical analysis. *Current Opinion in Clinical Nutrition and Metabolic Care* **8** (2), 171–175.

Woien, H. & Bjork, T. (2006) Nutrition of the critically ill patient and effects of implementing a nutritional support algorithm in ICU. *Journal of Clinical Nursing* **15** (2), 168–177.

Wolfe, B., Ryder, M., Nishikawa, R. *et al.* (1986) Complications of parenteral nutrition. *American Journal of Surgery* **152**, 93–99.

Woodcock, N. & MacFie, J. (2004) Optimal nutritional support. *Proceedings of the Nutrition Society* **63** (3), 451–452.

Woodrow, P. (2000) Intensive Care Nursing: *A Framework for Practice*. Routledge, London.

Monitoring Temperature

12

INTRODUCTION

The body can only function effectively within a narrow temperature range (Trim, 2005). Any significant changes in temperature, either a rise or a fall, can lead to life-threatening complications. As a critically ill patient can experience wide fluctuations in temperature, close temperature monitoring is paramount.

Monitoring the temperature in the critically ill patient is a vital yet often neglected part of the management of the critically ill patient (Andrews & Nolan 2006). As well as depressing organ function, hypothermia causes coagulopathy, increases blood loss and increases adrenergic responses which can increase morbidity (Andrews & Nolan 2006). Rewarming patients can cause cardiovascular instability.

Close monitoring of the temperature is also important if the patient has a condition that affects basal metabolic rate, e.g. thyrotoxicosis, is susceptible to infection, e.g. neutropenic, already has a local or systemic infection, is receiving a blood transfusion or is in the postoperative phase.

The aim of this chapter is to understand the principles of monitoring temperature.

LEARNING OBJECTIVES

At the end of this chapter the reader will be able to:

❏ discuss the factors *influencing* body temperature
❏ discuss the methods of *measuring* temperature
❏ discuss the physiological effects of *hypothermia*
❏ outline the *monitoring priorities* of a patent with *hypothermia*

❏ discuss the *physiological effects* of hyperthermia
❏ outline the *monitoring priorities* of a patient with *hyperthermia*

FACTORS INFLUENCING BODY TEMPERATURE

The normal body temperature is usually between 36 and 37.5°C, regardless of the environmental temperature (Trim 2005). Temperature is regulated by the thermoregulatory centre in the hypothalamus through various physiological mechanisms, e.g. sweating, dilation/constriction of peripheral blood vessels and shivering.

The body's core temperature is usually the highest, while the skin's is the coolest. Core temperature represents the balance between the heat generated by body tissues during metabolic activity, especially of the liver and muscles, and heat lost during various *mechanisms* (Mallett & Dougherty 2000).

There are four mechanisms of heat loss (Tappen & Andre 1996):

- *radiation*: flow of heat from a higher temperature (the body) to a lower temperature (environment surrounding the body)
- *convection*: heat transfer by flow or movement of air
- *conduction*: heat transfer due to direct contact with cooler surfaces
- *evaporation*: perspiration, respiration and breaks in skin integrity

There are several factors that can cause a fluctuation in temperature, including:

- The body's *circadian rhythms*: temperature is higher in the evening than the morning (Brown 1990), the difference can be as much as 1.5°C (Minor & Waterhouse 1981). If temperature is being recorded every 4–6 hours, the optimum time for detecting a pyrexia is probably between 7 and 8 pm (Angerami 1980).
- *Ovulation*.
- *Exercise* and *eating* can cause a rise in temperature (Marieb 1998).
- *Old age*: there is an increased sensitivity to the cold and there is generally a lower body temperature.
- *Illness*.

METHODS OF MEASURING TEMPERATURE

The traditional method of using oral/rectal mercury thermometers is now seldom used (Kelly *et al.* 2001). Mercury is covered by the Control of Substances Hazardous to Health Regulations (COSHH) (1999) and its vapour is neurotoxic (Woodrow 2000). In addition, although rectal temperature is closest to core temperature (Schmitz *et al.* 1994), it is unreliable in the critically ill patient because hypotension and gut ischaemia reduce the blood supply to the rectum (Holtzclaw 1992) and the measurement is influenced by the contents in the rectum.

There are, however, several reliable methods of measuring body temperature using electronic devices. These devices are fast, safe and some can provide continuous measurements of temperature (Tortora & Grabowski 1996). A selection will now be described in more detail.

Tympanic thermometers

The tympanic membrane shares the same carotid blood supply as the hypothalamus (Klein *et al.* 1993). Measurement of tympanic membrane temperature should therefore reflect core temperature (Woodrow 2000).

The tympanic thermometer (Fig. 12.1), which uses infrared light to detect thermal radiation (Woodrow 2000), is designed for intermittent use, offering a 'one-off' digital reading.

Care should be taken when using the tympanic thermometer, as poor technique can render the measurement inaccurate. Temperature differences between the opening of the ear canal and the tympanic membrane can be as much as 2.8°C (Hudak *et al.* 1998). To ensure the temperature measurements are accurate, the tympanic thermometer probe should be positioned to fit snugly in the ear canal. This will prevent ambient air at the opening of the ear canal from entering it, resulting in a false low temperature measurement (Jevon & Jevon 2001). Ear canal size, wax, operator technique and the patient's position can affect the accuracy of the measurements (Knies, 2003).

Chemical dot thermometers

Chemical dot thermometers are flexible polystyrene strips with a temperature sensor at one end, designed for single oral/axilla use. However their accuracy has been questioned (Erickson *et al.*

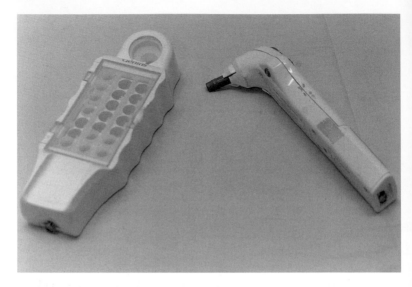

Fig. 12.1 Tympanic thermometer.

Best practice – tympanic temperature monitoring

Use the same ear for consecutive measurements
Install a new disposable probe cover for each measurement
Ensure thermometer probe is positioned snugly in the external
 auditory meatus
Aim the thermometer towards the tympanic membrane
Measure the patient's temperature following manufacturer's
 instructions
Consider the temperature reading alongside other systemic
 observations and overall condition of the patient
Store the thermometer following manufacturer's instructions
(Jevon & Jevon 2001)

1996). These thermometers are unsuitable in patients with hypothermia because their temperature range is restricted to 35.5–40.4°C (O'Toole 1997).

If the oral route is used, the strip should be placed in the sublingual pocket of tissue at the base of the tongue, which is close to the thermoreceptors which respond rapidly to changes in core temperature (Marinin & Wheeler 1997). It is important to ensure that the strip is placed in the sublingual pocket and not in the area under the front of the tongue because there may be a difference in temperature of up to 1.7°C between the two areas (Dougherty & Lister 2004).

Oral temperature measurements can be affected by the temperature of ingested foods and fluids and by the muscular activity of chewing (Dougherty & Lister 2004). In addition a respiratory rate of >18 breaths per minute will reduce core temperature values (Marieb 1998).

The axilla is an alternative route for temperature monitoring if the oral route is unsuitable, e.g. in a convulsive patient. However it can be difficult to obtain an accurate and reliable measurement because the site is not close to a major blood vessel and the surface temperature of the skin can be affected by the environment (Woollens 1996). If the axilla is used, the strip should be placed in the centre of the armpit with the patient's arm positioned firmly against the side of the chest. As the temperature can vary between arms, the same site should be used for serial measurements (Howell 1972).

Regardless of what site is used for temperature measurements, the same one should be consistently used, because switching between different sites can produce measurements that are both misleading and difficult to interpret (Dougherty & Lister 2004).

Oesophageal/nasopharangeal probes

The oesophageal probe should be accurately positioned in the lower quarter of the oesophagus (Aun 1997). The nasopharangeal temperature can be affected by air leaking around the tracheal tube. Both probes can be interfaced with the patient monitoring system, thus offering an accurate and continuous reading.

Bladder probe

Bladder and pulmonary artery temperature correlate well (Bartlett 1996) and because most critically ill patients require a urinary catheter, this method of measuring body temperature avoids additional invasive equipment. A thermocouple attached to the distal end of the catheter can interface with the patient monitoring system and offer continuous temperature measurements. This method of temperature measurement is considered to be very reliable (Lefrant *et al*. 2003).

Pulmonary artery catheter

Although the pulmonary artery catheter is the gold standard for temperature measurement (Fulbrook 1993), it is highly invasive and its sole use for temperature measurements cannot be justified. However if one is inserted, the thermistor sited in the distal end can interface with the patient's monitoring system and can provide continuous temperature measurements.

PHYSIOLOGICAL EFFECTS OF HYPOTHERMIA

Hypothermia, defined as a core temperature of <35°C (Trim 2005), can occur when the body loses too much heat or cannot maintain its normothermic state. There are several risk factors (Table 12.1). Table 12.2 shows the various signs and symptoms of hypothermia at different levels of temperature.

Table 12.1 Risk factors for hypothermia.

Children
Elderly people
Poor accommodation
Malnourishment
Exposure to a cold environment
Burns
Overdose of medications that lead to coma and immobility
Medications, e.g. benzodiazepines, morphine, barbiturates and vasodilators
Underlying illness, e.g. hypothyroidism
Alcohol abuse
Surgery

Adapted from Kelly *et al*. 2001.

Table 12.2 Signs and symptoms of hypothermia at different levels of temperature.

Temperature	Signs and symptoms
37.6°C	'Normal' rectal temperature
37°C	'Normal' oral temperature
36°C	Increased metabolic rate to attempt to balance heat loss
35°C	Shivering maximum at this temperature; hyper-reflexia, dysarthria, delayed cerebration
34°C	Patients usually responsive and with normal blood pressure; lower limit compatible with continued exercise
33–31°C	Retrograde amnesia, consciousness clouded, blood pressure difficult to obtain, pupils dilated, most shivering ceases
30–28°C	Progressive loss of consciousness, increased muscular rigidity, slow pulse and respiration, cardiac arrhythmias develop if heart irritated
27°C	Voluntary motion lost along with pupillary light reflex, deep tendon and skin reflexes; appears dead
26°C	Victims seldom conscious
25°C	Ventricular fibrillation may appear spontaneously
24–21°C	Pulmonary oedema develops (100% mortality in shipwreck victims in World War II)
20°C	Heart standstill
18°C	Lowest adult accidental hypothermic patient with recovery
17°C	Isoelectric EEG
15.2°C	Lowest infant accidental hypothermic patient with recovery
9°C	Lowest artificially cooled hypothermic patient with recovery
4°C	Monkeys revived successfully
1–7°C	Rats and hamsters revived successfully

Reproduced by kind permission of Cambridge University Press from Skinner *et al.* 1997.

Sometimes hypothermia is intentionally induced, e.g. during some cardiac surgery, either by heat exchange through a heart/lung machine or by surface cooling using ice. The aim is to reduce oxygen and metabolic demands, thus protecting the vital organs during low blood flow periods (Foldy & Gorman 1989).

When monitoring a patient with hypothermia it is important to understand the physiological effects it has on the various systems in the body. The main effects of hypothermia on the bodily systems are detailed below.

Cardiovascular system

Initially there is sympathetic stimulation which increases heart rate, blood pressure and cardiac output. However with increasing hypothermia there is progressive cardiovascular depression leading to a reduction in tissue perfusion and oxygenation (Oh 1997) and cardiac arrhythmias, e.g. bradycardia, atrial fibrillation and ventricular fibrillation, can become a problem (Resuscitation Council UK 2006). Rough movement and activity should be avoided as this can precipitate a cardiopulmonary arrest. Sometimes the patient's pulse may be difficult to detect.

Respiratory system

Following an initial reflex stimulation of respiration, there is a progressive decrease in respiratory rate, tidal volume and minute volume (Oh 1997; Chan *et al.* 1998) leading to hypoxaemia and hypoxia. Sometimes the patient's respirations may be difficult to detect (Resuscitation Council UK 2006).

Neurological system

Cerebral blood flow reduces at a rate of 7% for each 1°C drop in temperature (Hudak *et al.* 1998) resulting in confusion, decreased reflexes, cranial nerve deficits and lack of voluntary motion. Increased blood viscosity, decreased oxygen availability, lack of shivering and muscle rigidity also develop (Kelly *et al.* 2001).

Renal system

In mild hypothermia (32–35°C) sympathetic activity leads to an increase in cardiac output resulting in a 'cold' diuresis. However, with progressive hypothermia, renal blood flow and glomerular filtrate fall. Sodium and water losses may be evident due to metabolic failure of renal tubules (Murphy 1998).

Gastrointestinal system
If the temperature is <34°C, gut motility decreases which can lead to vomiting and malabsorption.

Metabolic system
Metabolic acidosis occurs due to accumulation of lactate and failure to secrete hydrogen ions. Hyperkalaemia resulting from the failure of membrane sodium/potassium pumps and hypoxic liver damage may also occur (Jackson 1998).

Endocrine system
Insulin secretion falls resulting in a failure of glucose utilisation and hyperglycaemia. If hypothermia is prolonged, glycogen stores can become depleted causing hypoglycaemia (Aun 1997).

Haematology
Potential complications include thrombocytopenia, coagulopathy and disseminated intravascular coagulation (Jackson 1998); splenic sequestration (breaking down or destruction) may also occur, resulting in a decrease in white cell and platelet formation (Aun 1997).

MONITORING PRIORITIES OF A PATIENT WITH HYPOTHERMIA
The monitoring priorities of a patient with hypothermia include:

- regular assessment of vital signs: airway, respirations, blood pressure, pulse and core temperature
- arterial blood gas analysis
- ECG monitoring to detect cardiac arrhythmias
- urine output measurements
- blood sugar measurements to detect hypoglycaemia
- neurological function observations

Monitoring during rewarming is also important. A patient warmer (Fig. 12.2) is commonly used for rewarming, though

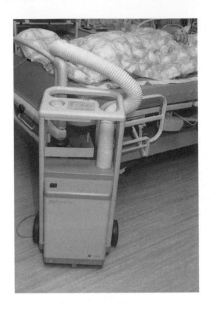

Fig. 12.2 Patient warmer.

other methods are available (Kelly *et al.* 2001). Rewarming should not exceed increases of 0.3–1.2°C per hour in cases of mild hypothermia; but rapid rewarming of >3°C per hour may be necessary if there are severe hypothermia and cardiovascular instability (Carson 1999).

Peripheral vasodilation may complicate active rewarming methods. This could induce hypotension and a further drop in core temperature, the latter increasing the risk of arrhythmias (Murphy 1998). 'Careful monitoring and supportive therapy during rewarming are mandatory' (Aun 1997).

PHYSIOLOGICAL EFFECTS OF HYPERTHERMIA
Sudden rises in temperature are often caused by infection. However, there are several other causes of hyperthermia, including:

- hyperthyroidism
- malignancy
- drug allergy
- damage to the central nervous system
- allergic reaction to blood transfusion
- heat stroke

(Dougherty & Lister 2004)

Pyrexia in response to infection is a protective mechanism. It inhibits bacterial and viral growth (Ganong 1995), promotes immunity and phagocytosis (Rowsey 1997) and, through hypermetabolism, promotes tissue repair (Woodrow 2000). Mild pyrexia is generally not treated.

However pyrexia and hypermetabolism can cause physiological stress (Woodrow 2000), e.g. a 13% increase in oxygen consumption with each 1°C rise in temperature (Nowak & Handford 1999), a rise in intracranial pressure (Morgan 1990) and cerebral damage (Closs 1992).

Severe hyperthermia or heat stroke is a temperature of >40°C (Aun 1997). It can be caused by MDMA ('ecstasy') (MacConnachie 1997), exposure to a high ambient temperature, vigorous activity and certain drugs (malignant hyperthermia). The main effects of severe hyperthermia on the bodily systems include:

- *cardiovascular system*: tachycardia, ECG changes and cardiac failure
- *respiratory system*: tachypnoea and respiratory alkalosis
- *neurological system*: confusion, delirium, convulsions and possibly coma
- *renal system*: loss of fluid and acute renal failure

(Jones *et al.* 2003)

MONITORING PRIORITIES OF A PATIENT WITH HYPERTHERMIA

Monitoring priorities of a patient with hyperthermia include:

- *regular assessment of vital signs*: airway, respirations, blood pressure, pulse and core temperature
- *arterial blood gas analysis*: particularly important if the patient has malignant hyperthermia, as acidosis is common

- *ECG monitoring*: to detect arrhythmias
- *urine output* measurements and strict fluid balance
- *blood sugar* measurements
- *neurological function* observations

In addition it is important to monitor any methods used to cool the patient. Core and skin temperature should be closely monitored to avoid overshoot hypothermia and rebound hyperthermia (Aun 1997).

Scenario

A 65-year-old lady was admitted with bronchopneumonia. She looked flushed and was hot to the touch. Her vital signs were BP 130/80, pulse 115, resps 25, tympanic temperature 34.4°C. The tympanic temperature reading is undoubtedly incorrect. What would you do?

There is probably an error with the equipment or technique. The lens on the thermometer was cleaned with a dry wipe. In addition, the end of the probe was placed in the external auditory meatus ensuring a snug fit. The tympanic temperature now showed 38.7°C which was more conducive with the patient's clinical condition.

CONCLUSION

A critically ill patient can experience wide fluctuations in body temperature. Severe hypothermia and hyperthermia can be life threatening. Close monitoring of temperature in the critically ill patient is therefore paramount. It is also paramount to understand the principles of monitoring a hypothermic and hyperthermic patient, particularly during rewarming or cooling procedures.

REFERENCES

Andrews, F. & Nolan, J. (2006) Critical care in the emergency department: monitoring the critically ill patient. *Emergency Medicine Journal* **23**, 561–564.

Angerami, E. (1980) Epidemiological study of body temperature in patients in a teaching hospital. *International Journal of Nursing Studies* **17**, 91–99.

Aun, C. (1997) Thermal disorders. In: T. Oh, ed. *Intensive Care Manual* 4th edn. Butterworth Heinemann, Oxford.

Bartlett, E. (1996) Temperature measurement: why and how in intensive care. *Intensive and Critical Care Nursing* **12** (1), 50–54.

Brown, S. (1990) Temperature taking – getting it right. *Nursing Standard* **5** (12), 4–5.

Carson, B. (1999) Successful resuscitation of a 44 year old man with hypothermia. *Journal of Emergency Nursing* **25** (5), 356–360.

Chan, E., Winston, B., Terada, L. & Parsons, P. (1998) *Bedside Critical Care Manual*. Hanley and Belfus, Philadelphia.

Closs, S. (1992) Patients' night-time pain, analgesia provision and sleep after surgery. *International Journal of Nursing Studies* **29** (4), 381–392.

Control of Substances Hazardous to Health Regulations (1999) The Stationery Office, London.

Doezema, D., Lunt, M. & Tandberg, D. (1995) Cerumen occlusion lowers infrared tympanic membrane temperature measurement. *Emergency Medicine* **2** (1), 17–19.

Dougherty, L. & Lister, S. (2004) eds *The Royal Marsden Hospital Manual of Clinical Nursing Procedures* 6th edn. Blackwell Publishing, Oxford.

Erickson, R., Meyer, L. & Woo, T. (1996) Accuracy of chemical dot thermometers in critically ill adults and young children. *Image – Journal of Nurse Scholarships* **28** (1), 23–28.

Foldy, S. & Gorman, J. (1989) Perioperative nursing care for congenital cardiac defects. *Critical Care Nursing Clinics of North America* **1**, 289–295.

Fulbrook, P. (1993) Core temperature measurement: a comparison of rectal, axillary and pulmonary artery temperature. *Intensive and Critical Care Nursing* **9** (4), 217–225.

Ganong, W. (1995) *Review of Medical Physiology* 17th edn. Prentice Hall, London.

Holtzclaw, B. (1992) The febrile response in critical care: state of the science. *Heart and Lung* **21** (5), 482–501.

Howell, T. (1972) Axillary temperature in aged women. *Age and Ageing* **1**, 250–254.

Hudak, C.M., Gallo, B.M. & Morton, P.G. (1998) *Critical Care Nursing: a Holistic Approach* 7th edn. Lippincott, New York.

Jackson, R. (1998) Physicial injury. In: P. Murphy, ed. *Handbook of Critical Care*. Science Press, London.

Jevon, P. & Jevon, M. (2001) Using a tympanic thermometer. *Nursing Times* **97** (9), 43–44.

Jones, G., Endacott, R. & Crouch, R. (2003) *Emergency Nursing Care*. Greenwich Medical Media Ltd, London.

Kelly, M., Ewens, B. & Jevon, P. (2001) Hypothermia management. *Nursing Times* **97** (9), 36–37.

Klein, D., Mitchell, C., Petrina, A. *et al.* (1993) A comparison of pulmonary artery, rectal and tympanic membrane temperature measurement in the ICU. *Heart and Lung* **22** (5), 435–441.

Knies, R. (2003) *Temperature measurement in acute care* www.enw.org/research-Thermometry.htm.

Lefrant, J., Muller, L. *et al.* (2003) Temperature measurement in intensive care patients: comparison of urinary bladder, oesophageal, rectal, axillary and inguinal methods versus pulmonary artery core method. *Intensive Care Medicine* **29**, 414–418.

MacConnachie, A. (1997) Ecstasy poisoning. *Intensive and Critical Care Nursing* **13** (6), 365–366.

Mallett, J. & Dougherty, L. (2000) eds *The Royal Marsden Hospital Manual of Clinical Nursing Procedures* 5th edn. Blackwell Science, Oxford.

Marieb, E. (1998) *Human Anatomy and Physiology* 4th edn. Benjamin Cummings, California.

Marinin, J. & Wheeler, A. (1997) *Medical Care Medicine* 2nd edn. Williams & Wilkins, London.

Minor, D. & Waterhouse, J. (1981) *Circadian Rhythms and the Human*. Wright, Bristol.

Morgan, S. (1990) A comparison of three methods of managing fever in the neurological patient. *Journal of Neuroscience Nursing* **22** (1), 19–24.

Murphy, P. (1998) ed. *Handbook of Critical Care*. Science Press, London.

Nowak, T. & Handford, A. (1999) *Essentials of Pathophysiology*. McGraw Hill, New York.

Oh, T. (1997) ed. *Intensive Care Manual* 4th edn. Butterworth Heinemann, Oxford.

O'Toole, S. (1997) Alternatives to mercury thermometers. *Professional Nurse* **12** (11), 783–786.

Resuscitation Council UK (2006) *Advanced Life Support* 5th edn. Resuscitation Council UK, London.

Rowsey, P. (1997) Pathophysiology of fever. Part 2: Relooking at cooling interventions. *Dimensions of Critical Care Nursing* **15** (5), 251–256.

Schmitz, T., Blair, N., Falk, M. *et al.* (1994) A comparison of five methods of temperature measurement in febrile intensive care patients. *American Journal of Intensive Care* **4** (4), 286–292.

Skinner, D.V., Swain, A., Robertson, C. & Rodney Peyton, J.W. (1997) *Cambridge Textbook of Accident and Emergency Medicine*. Cambridge University Press, Cambridge.

Tappen, R. & Andre, S. (1996) Inadvertent hypothermia in elderly surgical patients. *AORN Journal* **63** (3), 639–644.

Tortora, G. & Grabowski, S. (1996) *Principles of Anatomy and Physiology* 8th edn. Harper Collins, Boston.

Trim, J. (2005) Monitoring temperature. *Nursing Times* **101** (20), 30–31.

Woodrow, P. (2000) *Intensive Care Nursing: A Framework for Practice*. Routledge, London.

Woollens, S. (1996) Temperature measurement devices. *Professional Nurse* **11** (8), 541–547.

Monitoring During Transport

13

INTRODUCTION

It is estimated that over 11 000 critically ill patients require inter-hospital transport each year (Intensive Care Society 1997; Mackenzie *et al.* 1997). The main reasons for interhospital transport include lack of ICU beds, specialists, diagnostic tools and therapeutic means (Gebremichael *et al.* 2000).

Interhospital transport imposes essential risk for critically ill patients (Markakis *et al.* 2006). Despite the large numbers of inter-hospital transfers, the provision of equipment still remains poor and potentially serious complications frequently occur (Intensive Care Society 1997; Bion *et al.* 1988). The quality and outcome of the transfer depends on the experience of the transfer team, meticulous clinical preparation and adequate monitoring facili-ties (Tan 1997). This same level of supervision and preparation is also required for intrahospital transfer of critically ill patients (Intensive Care Society 1997). *Transport of the Critically Ill Adult Patient*, published by the Intensive Care Society (1997), makes recommendations for the organisation and clinical provision of transfers.

The aim of this chapter is to understand the principles of moni-toring a critically ill patient during transport.

LEARNING OBJECTIVES

At the end of the chapter the reader will be able to:

❏ list the possible *reasons* for transporting a critically ill patient, both within a hospital and from one hospital to another
❏ discuss the potential *problems* and *hazards* associated with transport
❏ discuss what *monitoring equipment* is required for transport
❏ discuss *what should be monitored* during transport

REASONS FOR TRANSPORT

Possible reasons for *intrahospital* transport of critically ill patients include:

- diagnostic and therapeutic procedures that can not be undertaken at the bedside, e.g. CT scan
- need for surgery
- transfer to ICU/HDU/CCU

Possible reasons for *interhospital* transport of critically ill patients include:

- non-clinical need, e.g. lack of an ICU bed
- requirement for specialist services, e.g. spinal unit
- requirement for specialist investigations, e.g. angiography
- requirement for specialist surgery, e.g. neurosurgery, cardiac surgery
- complex organ support
- social reasons, e.g. transfer to a hospital nearer to the patient's home

POTENTIAL PROBLEMS AND HAZARDS ASSOCIATED WITH TRANSPORT

Mortality rates during transport are remarkably low (<1%) (Hinds & Watson 1996). However, it is still potentially hazardous to transport a critically ill patient, particularly if intensive haemodynamic and respiratory support is required or if it is undertaken by unqualified or inexperienced staff (Bion *et al.* 1988).

The transport of critically ill patients can result in physiological deterioration (Waddell *et al.* 1975; Gentleman & Jennett 1981). The patient may be unable to tolerate lifting, tipping, abrupt movements, vibration and acceleration/deceleration (Lawler 2000). Accelerational forces and vertical movements can cause cardiovascular instability, particularly in patients who are hypovolaemic or vasodilated due to sepsis, drugs or sedation (Hinds & Watson 1996).

Significant changes in intracranial pressure can be induced by transport, e.g. placing a patient in the head down position when loading on to the ambulance can exacerbate intracranial hypertension (Hinds & Watson 1996). Helicopter transfer may be less hazardous to a critically ill patient, particularly if flown feet first, as this will result in a slightly head-up position during acceleration and a slightly head-down position during deceleration. This may minimise the changes in cardiovascular function and intracranial pressure often associated with transport (Kee *et al.* 1992).

An ambulance is probably the worst environment to care for a critically ill patient (Figs 13.1 and 13.2). Space limitations, movement, noise, power sources and lighting can all impose restrictions. Movement of the vehicle can make the performance of even the most routine medical and nursing procedures difficult. A particularly common problem is motion sickness, both for the patient and the staff.

Noise and daylight may render monitors and their alarms unreadable and inaudible. Ambulances rely on battery sources for electrical power. Consequently hospital-based equipment which needs alternating current (a.c.) can only be used with its own power source or an a.c./d.c. converter.

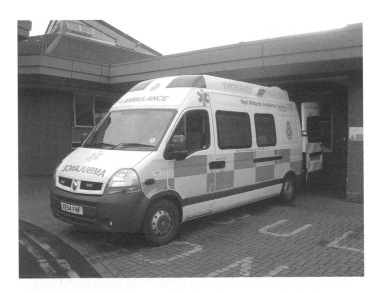

Fig. 13.1 Paramedic ambulance: the most common means of land transport.

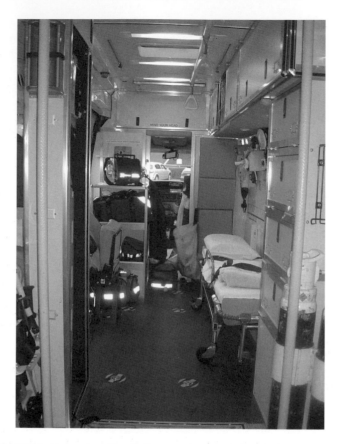

Fig. 13.2 Inside a paramedic ambulance.

Untoward occurrences, including accidental extubation, battery failure, loss of intravenous access and abrupt cessation of vasoactive or sedative agents, are not uncommon. In fact approximately 11–34% of all transports experience equipment problems and mishaps (Smith *et al*. 1990; Carson & Drew 1994; Evans & Winslow 1995).

Hazards associated with air transport

The hazards encountered with air transport are dependent to a degree on the mode of transport (helicopter or aeroplane) and can be summarised as follows:

- *Expansion of gas in closed cavities*: as atmospheric pressure falls with increasing altitude, the volume occupied by gas rises; clinically this will result in trapped gases expanding. This will exacerbate a pneumothorax. In addition air in a tracheal tube cuff is susceptible to these changes; either gently fill the cuff with normal saline or continuously monitor the cuff pressure during altitude changes.
- *Fluid loss*: a fall in atmospheric pressure can cause fluid to extravasate from the intravascular to the interstitial space resulting in oedema, hypotension and tachycardia; further, the effects of dehydration can be exacerbated (Hinds & Watson 1996).
- *Hypoxia*: increasing altitude causes a fall in the partial pressure of oxygen which can lead to a fall in alveolar oxygen and hypoxia.
- *Temperature control*: heating in helicopters can be particularly difficult. In addition the patient may be exposed to the environment when being transferred to and from the aircraft.
- *Noise*: will cause sensory deprivation; in particular helicopter noise can interfere with monitoring, especially audible warning devices (Kee *et al.* 1992).
- *Vibration*: can make monitoring difficult and can cause problems with gravity-dependent intravenous fluid administration.
- *Visibility*: may be reduced; this together with the noise can make monitoring even more difficult; visual alarms may be obscured.
- *Unfamiliar environment*: can be stressful for staff.

PATIENT MONITORING EQUIPMENT REQUIRED FOR TRANSPORT

Determining what monitoring equipment should be taken will depend on the condition of the patient and the available resources on the mode of transport. Any equipment taken should be:

- lightweight, yet durable and robust
- restrained, yet easily accessible
- regularly checked (Gilligan 1997)
- battery powered if electrical (with battery life display)

Ideally equipment should have both audible and visual alarms. A small versatile portable monitor such as a Propaq (Fig. 13.3) is invaluable. Depending on what is required, recordings of ECG, oxygen saturation, non-invasive blood pressure, temperature, invasive pressures and capnography can be taken. Capnography is recommended as a mandatory requirement by the Intensive Care Society (1997).

Infusion pumps (Fig. 13.4) and appropriate medications should be available. In particular it is important to ensure that essential infusions, e.g. vasoactive drugs, do not run out during transfer.

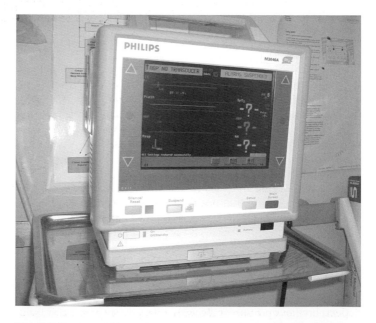

Fig. 13.3 Propaq portable monitor.

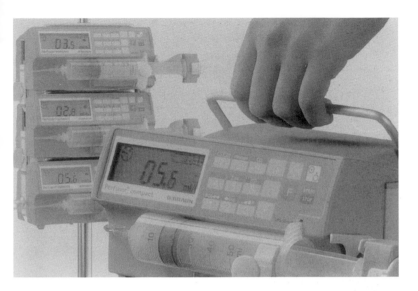

Fig. 13.4 Infusion pumps.

Although a mobile phone should ideally be available to help with communications, any possible effect on monitoring equipment should be checked. If air transport is being undertaken, *always* check with the pilot before using a mobile phone, as mobiles can interfere with aircraft navigation and avionics.

MONITORING DURING TRANSFER

The standard of care and monitoring during transport, which will depend on the individual needs of the patient, should be maintained at the same level as on the ICU. The Intensive Care Society (1997) makes the following recommendations:

- *Arterial oxygenation, ECG, and arterial pressure* should be monitored in every patient.
- *Invasive arterial monitoring* is preferable to non-invasive as the latter is sensitive to motion.
- *Central venous pressure, pulmonary artery wedge pressure or intracranial pressure* may be required in some patients; interpretation

may, however, be difficult in a moving ambulance and treatment is therefore difficult to control.

- If the patient is being *mechanically ventilated* the oxygen supply and airway pressure should be monitored; a means for detecting disconnection should be established (one third of hospitals do not have a ventilator disconnector alarm) (Knowles *et al.* 1999).
- *End tidal CO₂ measurement* is desirable particularly in patients with cerebral injury regardless of the cause, though fewer than 50% of hospitals have the facility to undertake this during transport (Knowles *et al.* 1999).
- *Temperature* should be monitored if it is abnormal, during long journeys or in cold weather.

Assessment of adequacy of ventilation is notoriously inaccurate in an ambulance (Knowles *et al.* 1999). There are now sophisticated portable ventilators which can maintain the most dependent patient, without compromising their respiratory rate, for limited periods of time (Fig. 13.5). These offer different modes and run on a battery, requiring only an oxygen cylinder source.

If parenteral nutrition is halted it is recommended to administer 10% glucose to avoid rebound hypoglycaemia (Gilligan 1997). The blood glucose should be closely monitored during transfer.

As well as monitoring the patient, it is also important to monitor the equipment continuously, particularly alarms. Intravenous infusions should also be closely monitored to ensure that the prescribed dose is being administered and that they have not run out.

Unskilled or inexperienced staff may not recognise or rectify problems (Braman *et al.* 1987). Experienced staff should be in attendance, e.g. a senior ICU nurse and an anaesthetist, who should have the necessary skills to manage any sudden and unexpected outcome.

CONCLUSION

Transporting a critically ill patient can be fraught with difficulties and is potentially hazardous. Therefore it is important to justify

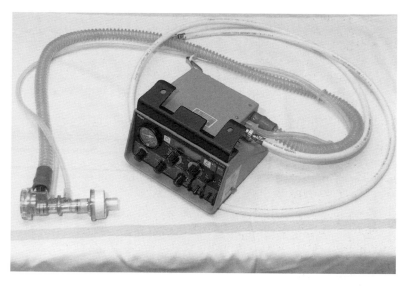

Fig. 13.5 Transport ventilator.

any transport whether it is intrahospital or interhospital. Knowledge of potential problems and hazards associated with transport is essential if patient monitoring during transport is to be undertaken accurately and effectively, thus minimising morbidity and mortality.

Risks are reduced when there are meticulous clinical preparation and appropriate equipment available for use, and when transfer is undertaken by experienced staff familiar with the transfer environment. The same level of supervision and preparation is also important when critically ill patients are transferred between departments within a hospital.

ACKNOWLEDGEMENT

Some text in this chapter has been reproduced, with kind permission, from Jevon, P. & Ewens, B. (2001) Care of patients on the move. *Nursing Times* **97** (4), 35–36.

REFERENCES

Bion, J.F., Wilson, I.H. & Taylor, P.A. (1988) Transporting critically ill patients by ambulance: audit by sickness scoring. *British Medical Journal* **296**, 170–174.

Braman, S., Dunn, S., Amico, C.A. & Millman, R.P. (1987) Complications of intrahospital transport in critically ill patients. *Annals of Internal Medicine* **107**, 469–473.

Carson, B. (1999) Successful resuscitation of a 44 year old man with hypothermia. *Journal of Emergency Nursing* **25** (5), 356–360.

Carson, K.J. & Drew, B.J. (1994) Electrocardiographic changes in critically ill adults during intrahospital transport. *Progress in Cardiovascular Nursing* **9** (4), 4–12.

Evans, A. & Winslow, E.H. (1995) Oxygen saturation and hemodynamic response in critically ill, mechanically ventilated adults during intrahospital transport. *American Journal of Critical Care* **4** (2), 106–111.

Gebremichael, M., Borg, U., Habashi, M. *et al.* (2000) Interhospital transport of the extremely ill patient: the mobile intensive care unit. *Critical Care Medicine* **28**, 79–85.

Gentleman, D. & Jennett, B. (1981) Hazards of inter-hospital transfer of comatose head-injured patients. *The Lancet* **1**, 853–855.

Gilligan, J. (1997) Transport of the critically ill. In: T. Oh, ed. *Intensive Care Manual* 4th edn. Butterworth-Heinemann, Oxford.

Hinds, C.J. & Watson, D. (1996) *Intensive Care, A Concise Textbook* 2nd edn. W.B. Saunders, London.

Intensive Care Society (1997) *Guidelines for the Transport of Critically Ill Patients.* Intensive Care Society, London.

Kee, S.S., Ramage, C.M.H., Mednel, P. & Bristow, A.S.E. (1992) Interhospital transfers by helicopter: the first 50 patients of the Care-light project. *Journal of the Royal Society of Medicine* **85**, 29–31.

Knowles, P.R., Bryden, P.C., Kishen, R. & Gwinnutt, C.L. (1999) Meeting the standards for interhospital transfer of adults with severe head injury in the United Kingdom. *Anaesthesia* **54** (3), 283–288.

Lawler, P.G. (2000) Transfer of critically ill patients: Part 1 – Physiological concepts. *Care of the Critically Ill* **16** (2), 61–65.

Lee, A., Lum, M.E., Beehan, S.J. & Hillman, K.M. (1996) Interhospital transfers: decision making in critical care areas. *Critical Care Medicine* **24** (4), 618–622.

Mackenzie, P.A., Smith, E.A. & Wallace, P.G.M. (1997) Transfer of adults between intensive care units in the United Kingdom: postal survey. *British Medical Journal* **314**, 455–456.

Markakis, C., Dalezios, M., Chatzicostas, C. *et al.* (2006) Evaluation of a risk score for interhospital transport of critically ill patients. *Emergency Medicine Journal* **23**, 313–317.

Smith, I., Fleming, S. & Cernaianu, A. (1990) Mishaps during transport from the intensive care unit. *Critical Care Medicine* **18** (2), 278–281.

Tan, T.K. (1997) Interhospital and intrahospital transfer of the critically ill patient. *Singapore Medical Journal* **36** (6), 244–248.

Waddell, G., Scott, P.D.R. & Lees, N.W. (1975) Effects of ambulance transport in critically ill patients. *British Medical Journal* **1**, 386–389.

14 | Record Keeping

INTRODUCTION

Good record keeping is a fundamental part of nursing (NMC 2005). An accurate written record detailing all aspects of patient monitoring is important, not only because it forms an integral part of the nursing management of the patient, but also because it can help to protect practitioners if defense of their actions is required. The Clinical Negligence Scheme for Trusts (CNST) also requires its members to maintain high standards of record keeping (Dimond 2005).

The aim of this chapter is to understand the principles of good record keeping, with specific reference to *Guidelines for Records and Record Keeping* (NMC 2005) (Fig. 14.1).

LEARNING OBJECTIVES

At the end of the chapter the reader will be able to:

❏ discuss the importance of good record keeping
❏ list the common deficiencies of record keeping
❏ outline the principles of good record keeping
❏ outline the importance of auditing records
❏ discuss the legal issues associated with record keeping

IMPORTANCE OF GOOD RECORD KEEPING

'Record keeping is an integral part of nursing, midwifery and health visiting practice. It is a tool of professional practice and one that should help the care process. It is not separate from this process and it is not an optional extra to be fitted in if circumstances allow.' (NMC 2005)

Good record keeping will help to protect the welfare of both the patient and practitioner by promoting:

- high standards of clinical care
- continuity of care
- better communication and dissemination of information between members of the inter-professional healthcare team
- the ability to detect problems, such as changes in the patient's condition at an early stage
- an accurate account of treatment and care planning and delivery

The quality of record keeping is also a reflection of the standard of nursing practice: good record keeping is an indication that the practitioner is professional and skilled while poor record keeping often highlights wider problems with the individual's practice (NMC 2005).

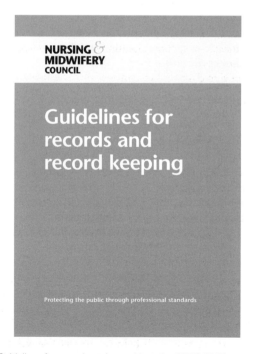

Fig. 14.1 *Guidelines for records and record keeping* (NMC 2005).

COMMON DEFICIENCIES IN RECORD KEEPING

Nearly every report published by the Health Service Commissioner (Health Service Ombudsman) following a complaint identifies examples of poor record keeping that have either hampered the care the patient has received or have made it difficult for healthcare professionals to defend their practice (Dimond 2005).

Common deficiencies in record keeping encountered include:

- absence of clarity
- failure to record action taken when a problem has been identified
- missing information
- spelling mistakes
- inaccurate records

(Dimond 2005)

PRINCIPLES OF GOOD RECORD KEEPING

There is a number of factors that underpin good record keeping. The patient's records should:

- be factual, consistent and accurate
- be updated as soon as possible after any recordable event
- provide current information on the care and condition of the patient
- be documented clearly and in such a way that the text cannot be erased
- be consecutive and accurately dated, timed and signed (including a printed signature)
- have any alterations and additions dated, timed and signed; all original entries should be clearly legible
- not include abbreviations, jargon, meaningless phrases, irrelevant speculation and offensive subjective statements
- still be legible if photocopied
- identify any problems identified and most importantly the action taken to rectify them

It is important to record all aspects of patient monitoring. Some observations will be recorded on the patient's observation charts (e.g. the ICU Observation Chart and the Standard Observation Chart, Fig. 14.2). Dates and times should be clearly visible and standard coloured ink should be used following local protocols. It is also important to ensure that an accurate record is made in the patient's notes. In particular it is important to include interventions and any response to the interventions.

Best practice – record keeping

Records must be:

factual
legible
clear
concise
accurate
signed
timed
dated

(Drew *et al.* 2000)

IMPORTANCE OF AUDITING RECORDS

Audit can play an important role in ensuring quality of health care. In particular it can help to improve the process of record keeping. By auditing records the standard can be evaluated and any areas for improvement and staff development identified. Audit tools should be developed at a local level to monitor the standards of record keeping.

Audit should primarily be aimed at serving the interests of the patient rather than the organisation (NMC, 2005). A system of peer review may also be of value. Whatever audit system is used, the confidentiality of patients' information applies to audit just as it does to record keeping.

LEGAL ISSUES ASSOCIATED WITH RECORD KEEPING

The patient's records are occasionally required as evidence before a court of law, by the Health Service Commissioner or in order to investigate a complaint at a local level. Sometimes they may be requested by the NMC's Fitness to Practice committees when investigating complaints related to misconduct. Care plans,

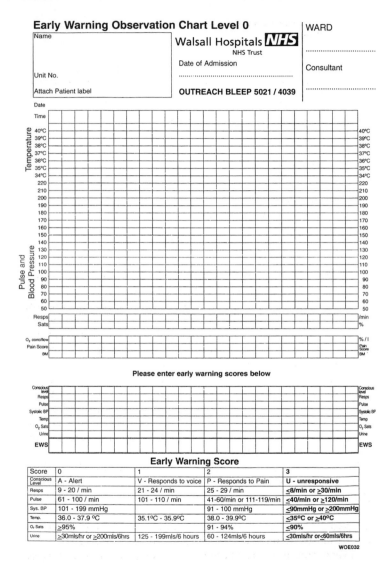

Early Warning Observation Chart Level 0

WARD

Name

Walsall Hospitals **NHS**
NHS Trust

Date of Admission

Consultant

Unit No.

Attach Patient label

OUTREACH BLEEP 5021 / 4039

Please enter early warning scores below

Early Warning Score

Score	0	1	2	3
Conscious Level	A - Alert	V - Responds to voice	P - Responds to Pain	**U - unresponsive**
Resps	9 - 20 / min	21 - 24 / min	25 - 29 / min	**≤8/min or ≥30/min**
Pulse	61 - 100 / min	101 - 110 / min	41-60/min or 111-119/min	**≤40/min or ≥120/min**
Sys. BP	101 - 199 mmHg		91 - 100 mmHg	**≤90mmHg or ≥200mmHg**
Temp.	36.0 - 37.9 °C	35.1°C - 35.9°C	38.0 - 39.9°C	**≤35°C or ≥40°C**
O₂ Sats	≥95%		91 - 94%	**≤90%**
Urine	≥30mls/hr or ≥200mls/6hrs	125 - 199mls/6 hours	60 - 124mls/6 hours	**≤30mls/hr or<60mls/6hrs**

WOE032

Fig. 14.2 Standard observation chart (Walsall Hospitals NHS Trust).

Notes   • = Calculate score EVERY time the observations are recorded
   < = less than
   > = greater than
   ≥ = the same or greater than
   ≤ = the same or less than
   • = If the score is three or above inform the nurse in charge who should follow the algorithm
   • = Urine output should be calculated according to body weight i.e. 0.5ml / kg/hr if weight known
      and from the preceding 6 hours
   • Score 1 - 2 repeat in 1 hour
   • ≥3 follow algorithm
   O_2 record in L / min if Hudson mask, O_2 % if variable mask i.e. venturi

Pain Assessment Tool
   1. **Comfortable**
   2. **Mild discomfort**
   3. **In pain**
   4. **In bad pain**
   5. **In very bad pain (excruciating pain)**

Fig. 14.2 *Continued* Explanatory notes to standard observation chart.

diaries and anything that makes reference to the patient's care may be required as evidence (NMC 2005).

What constitutes a legal document is often a cause for concern. Any document requested by the court becomes a legal document (Dimond 1994), e.g. nursing records, medical records, radiographs, laboratory reports, observation charts; in fact any document which may be relevant to the case.

If any of the documents are missing, the writer of the records may be cross-examined as to the circumstances of their disappearance (Dimond 1994). 'Medical records are not proof of the truth of the facts stated in them but the maker of the records may be called to give evidence as to the truth as to what is contained in them' (Dimond 1994).

The approach to record keeping which courts of law adopt tends to be that if it is not recorded, it has not been undertaken (NMC 2005). Professional judgment is required when deciding what is relevant and what needs to be recorded, particularly if the patient's clinical condition is apparently unchanging and no record has been made of the care that has been delivered.

A registered nurse has both a professional and a legal duty of care. Consequently when keeping records it is important to be able to demonstrate that:

- a comprehensive nursing assessment of the patient has been undertaken including care that has been planned and provided
- relevant information is included together with any measures that have been taken in response to changes in the patient's condition
- the duty of care owed to the patient has been honoured and that no acts or omissions have compromised the patient's safety
- arrangements have been made for ongoing care of the patient

The registered nurse is also accountable for any delegation of record keeping to members of the multi-professional team who are not registered practitioners. For example, if record keeping is delegated to a pre-registration student nurse or a healthcare assistant, competence to perform the task must be ensured and adequate supervision provided. All such entries must be countersigned.

The Access to Health Records Act 1990 gives patients the right of access to their manually maintained health records which were made after 1 November 1991. The Data Protection Act 1998 gives patients the right to access their computer-held records. The Freedom of Information Act 2000 grants the rights to anyone to all information that is not covered by the Data Protection Act 1998 (NMC 2005).

Sometimes it is necessary to withhold information if it could affect the physical or mental well-being of the patient or if it would breach another patient's confidentiality (NMC 2005). If the decision to withhold information is made, justification for doing so must be clearly recorded in the patient's notes.

CONCLUSION

When monitoring a critically ill patient it is important to ensure good record keeping. Good record keeping is both the product of good teamwork and an important tool in promoting high-quality health care.

REFERENCES

Dimond, B. (1994) *Legal Aspects in Midwifery*. Books for Midwives. Midwifery Press, Cheshire.

Dimond, B. (2005) Exploring common deficiencies that occur in record keeping. *British Journal of Nursing* **14** (10), 568–570.
Drew, D., Jevon, P. & Raby, M. (2000) *Resuscitation of the Newborn.* Butterworth Heinemann, Oxford.
NMC (2005) *Guidelines for Records and Record Keeping.* NMC, London.

Index